Practical Therapeutics
for the Older P

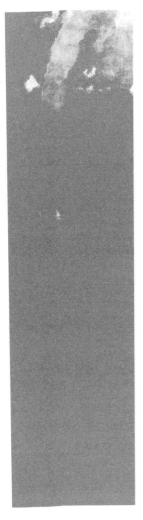

2003

2004

2005

To Daniel and Robert

Practical Therapeutics for the Older Patient

DENIS O'MAHONY

and

UNA MARTIN
The University of Birmingham, UK

JOHN WILEY & SONS

Chichester • New York • Weinheim
Brisbane • Singapore • Toronto

Copyright © 1999 John Wiley & Sons Ltd, Baffins Lane, Chichester, West Sussex
PO19 1UD, England

National 01243 779777 International (+44) 1243 779777
e-mail (for orders and customer service enquiries):
cs-books@wiley.co.uk
Visit our Home Page on http://www.wiley.co.uk
or http://www.wiley.com

Other Wiley Editorial Offices

John Wiley & Sons, Inc., 605 Third Avenue, New York, NY 10158-0012, USA

WILEY-VCH Verlag GmbH, Pappelallee 3, D-69469 Weinheim, Germany

Jacaranda Wiley Ltd, 33 Park Road, Milton, Queensland 4064, Australia

John Wiley & Sons (Asia) Pte Ltd, Clementi Loop #02-01, Jim Xing Distripark,
Singapore 129809

John Wiley & Sons (Canada) Ltd, 22 Worcester Road, Rexdale, Ontario
M9W 1L1, Canada

Library of Congress Cataloging-in-Publication Data

Practical therapeutics for the older patient / Denis O'Mahony and Una Martin.
    p.   cm.
  Includes bibliographical references and index.
  ISBN 0-471-98594-5 (pbk.)
  1. Geriatric pharmacology.   I. O'Mahony, Denis.   II. Martin, Una.
RC953.7.P724   1999
618.97'061—dc21   98-36751
                                                                           CIP

British Library Cataloguing in Publication Data

A catalogue record for this book is available from the British Library
ISBN 0-471-98594-5 (paper)

Typeset in 10/11½ pt Times from the authors' disks by Techset Composition Ltd, Salisbury,
Wiltshire
Printed and bound in Great Britain by Bookcraft (Bath) Ltd, Midsomer Norton, Somerset

2 6 JAN 1999

Contents

Foreword

Older people have much to gain from modern medicine. Drugs are becoming more effective and specific. Developments in surgery and anaesthetics are making operative interventions less challenging to frail older people. In terms of saving lives, treatments can be more effective for older than for younger people. Unfortunately, because of perversities in the requirements for licensing and evaluation of new drugs, older people are all too often excluded from trials of treatments from which they could benefit. Now that age-based rationing is being covertly practised and, by a noisy minority, advocated, it is important to establish the principle that where information is lacking, the burden of evidence lies on those who wish to urge that treatments that are effective for the young are not at least as effective for the old. There are anxieties, however, that older people may be at risk of undesirable side-effects from some interventions, not simply because they are old but because they may have cryptic comorbidity or physiological impairments. In extrapolating from young to old, therefore, a doctor needs to understand the mechanisms of treatment effects and so to know what precautions are appropriate and what hazards should be looked for. In its review of therapeutics for older people, this book summarizes what is known and what is reasonable to assume in responding to the needs of the increasing numbers of older patients presenting in general practice and hospital. Unique in its comprehensive range and succinct format, it deserves a favoured place on surgery desks and in white-coat pockets.

John Grimley Evans

Acknowledgements

The authors would like to express their thanks to the following colleagues for their expert help and advice in the preparation of this volume: Professor Martin Kendall, Dr Jon Townend, Dr Alistair Main, Dr Heather Morrison, Dr Peter Bentham, Dr Fidelma Dunne, Dr Bob Allan, Dr Paresh Jobanputra, Dr Frances Stafford, Dr Nigel Bailey, Dr Mark Temple, Ms Elizabeth Eagling, Dr Jim Murray, Dr Graham Stewart, Dr Christina Faull and Mrs Carol Dealey. Special thanks go to Professor Sir John Grimley Evans for encouraging the original idea for this book. We also owe our gratitude to the production team at John Wiley & Sons Ltd, in particular Mr Michael Osuch, Dr Lewis Derrick and Ms Laila Grieg-Gran for their support with bringing this publication to completion.

Finally, we acknowledge the constant support and patience of our spouses and families throughout the writing of this book.

Chapter 1

Central Issues in Geriatric Pharmacology

Older people constitute 18% of the population but receive 45% of all prescriptions. Unfortunately, patients are more likely to have problems with their medicines as they grow older. The increased number and frequency of disease processes with old age means that elderly patients are more likely to be on medication and often are taking several drugs at once. In addition, over 70% of 'over-the-counter' medicines are purchased by elderly people. It is not surprising that up to 10% of hospital admissions in this age group may result from an adverse drug reaction. Compounding the problems of high prescription rates and polypharmacy are changes in drug disposition, increased drug interactions, and difficulties with compliance in this age group.

1.1 PHARMACOKINETICS AND PHARMACODYNAMIC CHANGES IN THE ELDERLY

Physiological changes occur with age which may alter the way the body deals with medication (Table 1.1). However, the consequences of changes in absorption, distribution and hepatic metabolism may be difficult to detect in routine clinical practice. By comparison, the reduced renal clearance of renally excreted drugs may be readily observed.

1.1.1 Absorption

Few drugs have significantly delayed rates of absorption in elderly patients. Bioavailability of drugs will be increased for some drugs that

Table 1.1   Pharmacokinetic changes with age

Total absorption unchanged for most drugs
Bioavailability increased for drugs with high presystemic clearance
Distribution of fat-soluble drugs increased
Increased free concentration of weakly acidic drugs
Reduced liver size and blood flow leads to reduced hepatic clearance
Reduced renal function causes reduced excretion of many drugs

undergo presystemic first-pass metabolism, such as propranolol and nifedipine, because of a decline in hepatic excretion.

1.1.2   Distribution

A decrease in lean body mass and a corresponding increase in adipose tissue occurs with age. The distribution of lipid-soluble drugs such as diazepam may increase and result in a prolonged action. Similarly, water-soluble drugs, such as ethanol and digoxin, result in higher initial plasma concentrations in older people for any given dose based on body weight. Although albumin levels also decrease, the change is minimal unless there is associated disease, immobility or poor nutrition. In these circumstances an increase in plasma free drug concentrations of weakly acidic drugs such as phenytoin may increase the amount of drug available to exert a therapeutic or toxic effect and plasma concentrations, which measure free and bound drug, may be misleading if used to guide dosing. On the other hand, plasma levels of alpha-1-acid glycoprotein increases with age and basic drugs such as lignocaine may be more protein bound than in young patients.

1.1.3   Metabolism

Clearance of drugs by the liver is dependent on the activity of its metabolic enzymes and on liver blood flow. Hepatic mass declines with age so metabolism of many drugs with low intrinsic clearance will be reduced due to a reduction in microsomal enzyme activity. The metabolic pathways involved comprise phase 1 reactions, which make the compound less lipophilic but still partly or fully active, and phase 2 conjugation reactions, which make the compound even more polar and so more easily excreted by the kidneys. Phase 1, but not phase 2, reactions may be reduced with age. The action of drugs such as diazepam which undergo phase 1 and then phase 2 metabolism may therefore be prolonged in the elderly. However, other benzodiazepines, such as lorazepam, undergo conjugation reactions only and so metabolism is unaltered with age. For drugs that have a very rapid rate of metabolism and consequently high excretion rates across the liver, the decline of hepatic blood flow of 35% which occurs in people over 65 years means a reduction in systemic and presystemic clearance. This may increase the effects of drugs such as propranolol, chloromethiazole and morphine.

1.1.4 Renal Excretion

Most polar drugs or drug metabolites are excreted by the kidney. There is a steady decline in glomerular filtration rate with normal ageing so that between the ages of 20 and 70 a person may have up to 50% reduction in renal function. Many drugs such as digoxin, atenolol or amiloride which are dependent on the kidney for elimination will accumulate to toxic levels in older people if given in the usual doses for younger adults. Furthermore, many drugs such as aminoglycosides, diuretics and non-steroidal anti-inflammatory drugs (NSAIDs) are more likely to affect the kidney adversely in this age group. In practice, it is this decline in renal function that is the major pharmacokinetic determinant of toxicity in elderly patients. The **Cockcroft formula** may be used at the bedside to estimate the creatinine clearance and is helpful when deciding whether a dose reduction is necessary.

$$\text{Creatinine clearance (male)}$$
$$= \frac{1.23 \times (140 - \text{age}) \times \text{body weight (kg)}}{\text{plasma creatinine } (\mu\text{mol/l})}$$

$$\text{Creatinine clearance (female)}$$
$$= \frac{1.03 \times (140 - \text{age}) \times \text{body weight (kg)}}{\text{plasma creatinine } (\mu\text{mol/l})}$$

The effect of a drug on its site of action alters with age. However, such pharmacodynamic changes may be difficult to quantify in the elderly, who may show both increased and decreased responsiveness to medication. For example, elderly people may have problems with antihypertensives for several reasons: altered homeostatic mechanisms due to impaired baroreceptor function may result in postural hypotension, a reduction in first-pass metabolism may result in higher concentrations of certain calcium antagonists and beta-blockers and higher baseline blood pressure readings may result in a greater reduction in blood pressure with angiotensin-converting enzyme (ACE) inhibitors, particularly after the first dose.

1.2 COMPLIANCE

Problems with compliance may occur in up to 50% of elderly people (Table 1.2). Poor communication between doctors and patients seems to be the major problem. Patients are frequently given inadequate instructions or may not be able to hear, see or understand them. They often have little knowledge about side-effects and may take the wrong dose at the wrong time or continue to take tablets which have been changed. Compliance also decreases with an increasing number of drugs prescribed and the complexity of the regimen. Undoubtedly, these

Table 1.2 Causes of impaired compliance in older people

Adverse drug effects
Poor doctor/patient relationship
Polypharmacy
Social isolation
Depression
Complex therapeutic regimens
Packaging and delivery device problems
Cognitive impairment

Reproduced from *Medication for Older People* 2nd edn, 1997, by permission of the Royal College of Physicians of London.

problems are made worse in elderly patients, where there may be a degree of mental or visual impairment or where the patient may not have the manual dexterity to open childproof containers or blister packs.

1.3 DRUG–DRUG INTERACTIONS

Polypharmacy and the use of over-the-counter (OTC) drugs increases the likelihood that drugs will interact with one another, resulting in enhanced or reduced efficacy or the appearance of a new effect. Studies continue to show that older people receive unnecessary polypharmacy and are the major users of OTC medications, the range of which has changed considerably in recent years. In addition to antacids, cough medicines and laxatives, many other drugs are now readily available including non-sedating antihistamines, topical corticosteroids, oral and topical NSAIDs, nicotine patches and H_2-receptor antagonists. Nearly three-quarters of older patients do not discuss their OTC medication with the general practitioner who then may not be alerted about potential risks of interactions between any prescribed and non-prescribed medication.

Drug–drug interactions often have a pharmacokinetic basis. The rate at which a drug is absorbed may be decreased by anticholinergics, which inhibit gastric emptying, or increased by metoclopramide, which speeds up gastric emptying. Antacids and cholestyramine may bind to digoxin in the gut and reduce its bioavailability by up to 30%. Few other interactions affect drug absorption to a clinically significant effect.

Drugs which undergo extensive first-pass metabolism may be affected by other drugs which compete for metabolism or alter liver blood flow. Although highly protein-bound drugs may displace one another from plasma proteins, the interaction is usually not clinically significant. On the other hand, drugs such as cimetidine may inhibit the liver metabolism of many drugs including, benzodiazepines, beta-blockers, tricyclic antidepressants, theophylline, phenytoin and warfarin, leading to toxicity. Liver enzyme inducers such as carbamazepine may reduce the efficacy of warfarin or dihydropyridine calcium channel blockers. Finally, one drug may interfere with the excretion of another in the kidney. Prolonged treatment with thiazides increases lithium resorption by up to 50%.

Drugs may also antagonize the effects of one another: NSAIDs may reduce the effect of antihypertensives by causing sodium retention; diuretics may increase digoxin toxicity by causing hypokalaemia and beta-blockers and verapamil may lead to myocardial depression, hypotension and heart block when taken in combination.

1.4   ADVERSE DRUG REACTIONS

Adverse drug reactions are common in elderly people, particularly if they have an acute illness. Approximately 1 in 10 patients over 60 are admitted to hospital because of an adverse drug reaction or develop one during their stay. Reporting rates of serious adverse drug reactions expressed per million first prescriptions also increase with age (Figure 1.1). There are two main categories of adverse reaction. Type A reactions are attributable to accentuation of a drug's known pharmacological action and are related to dose. As such they are common and relatively predictable. Type B reactions are idiosyncratic, unrelated to dose, frequently unpredictable and of unknown mechanism. There is often a genetic or allergic basis to the reactions and although they are uncommon they tend to be more serious than type A reactions.

The most common adverse drug reactions are those affecting the gastrointestinal, central nervous and cardiovascular systems. For example, several studies have identified age as a clear positive risk factor for gastrointestinal bleeding due to NSAIDs. Elderly people are also more susceptible to the sedative effects of many centrally acting drugs such as the benzodiazepines. The wider implications for morbidity include an increase in hip fractures in elderly people taking hypnotics. With many drugs the time of greatest susceptibility to adverse drug reactions is during the first few days of treatment so an initial period of vigilance is particularly important in this age group.

1.5   INAPPROPRIATE PRESCRIBING

Therapy is inappropriate when given for an incorrect diagnosis or where the drug poses a high risk of adverse effects with little likelihood of benefit. Inappropriate prescribing is a particular problem for individuals living in long-term continuing care accommodation where over 90% of patients receive medication and polypharmacy is frequent. The use of sedation is particularly common and results in a high incidence of over-sedation, confusion and anticholinergic effects. In a study of private nursing homes in the UK nearly half the patients were prescribed major tranquillizers or benzodiazepines of whom only 12% had a clear indication for such therapy. Inappropriate prescribing is particularly likely when a symptom is treated without making an accurate diagnosis, e.g. the use of levodopa for phenothiazine-induced Parkinsonism.

1.6 REDUCING PROBLEMS CAUSED BY DRUGS

The Royal College of Physicians has issued updated guidelines to help doctors prescribe safely for the elderly. The principal recommendations are listed in Table 1.3.

1.7 GOLDEN RULES OF GOOD PRESCRIBING IN THE ELDERLY

(i) Before starting treatment with any drug the doctor must ensure that a correct diagnosis has been made and that a careful drug history has been taken.

(ii) A smaller dose than normal may be appropriate to start with and the duration of treatment must be specified.

(iii) Compliance may be improved in several ways (Table 1.3), including simplifying therapeutic regimens, explaining why the drug(s) are necessary and what adverse effects may occur.

(iv) Before starting a new drug the doctor should ensure that a new symptom is not an adverse effect of one of the drugs already taken.

(v) Medication should be clearly labelled and dispensed in containers that are easily opened.

(vi) Relatives may need to be involved with ensuring compliance.

(vii) Regular review of long-term therapy is essential. Pharmacists may provide compliance aids such as the Dosett box, which divides weekly amounts of drugs into separate timed daily doses. Finally, many drugs are particularly hazardous in the elderly and should be

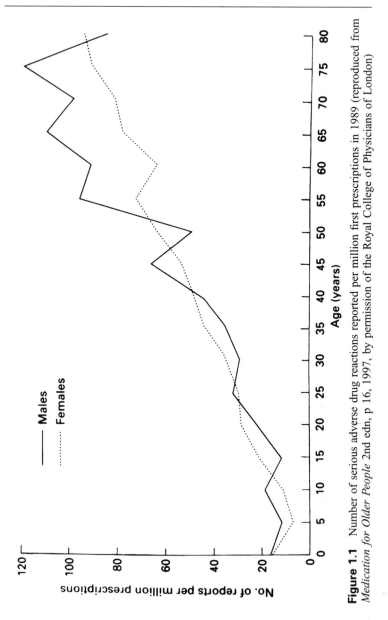

Figure 1.1 Number of serious adverse drug reactions reported per million first prescriptions in 1989 (reproduced from *Medication for Older People* 2nd edn, p 16, 1997, by permission of the Royal College of Physicians of London)

Table 1.3   Reducing problems caused by drugs

Make a diagnosis before prescribing
Check drug history
Use as few drugs as possible
Start with smaller dose
Keep dose regimen simple
Specify duration of treatment
Explain why drug is necessary
Describe possible adverse effects
Use clearly labelled, easily opened containers
Check inhaler technique
Consider compliance aids
Involve relatives or carers if necessary
Maintain adequate supervision of long-term medication

Reproduced from *Medication for Older People* 2nd edn, 1997, by permission of the Royal College of Physicians of London.

avoided if possible, particularly psychotropics, opioid analgesics and drugs with powerful hypotensive effects.

FURTHER READING

Cockcroft DW, Gault MH. Prediction of creatinine clearance from serum creatinine. *Nephron* 1976; 16:31–41.

Jackson GA, McGrath AM. Survey of neuroleptic prescribing in residents of nursing homes in Glasgow. *Br Med J* 1996; 312:611–612.

Montamat SC, Cusack BJ, Vestal RE. Management of drug therapy in the elderly. *N Engl J Med* 1989; 321:303–309.

Royal College of Physicians of London Working Party. *Medication for Older People*, 2nd edn. RCP, London, 1997.

Chapter 2

Cardiovascular Disorders

2.1 PREVENTIVE CARDIOVASCULAR MEDICINE IN OLD AGE

Cardiovascular disease is the main cause of death in Western countries. Of these deaths about 50% are caused by coronary heart disease and 25% by stroke. Mortality and morbidity from cardiovascular disease are largely preventable in elderly people. The three major modifiable risk factors are hypertension, hypercholesterolaemia and smoking.

2.1.1 Hypertension

Several multicentre prospective studies have shown that the higher the systolic or diastolic blood pressure (BP) the greater the cardiovascular morbidity and mortality rates. In the elderly, isolated systolic hypertension increases the risk of cardiovascular death by 2 to 5 times and the risk of stroke by 2.5 times. Respective 40% and 20% reductions in stroke and coronary heart disease events can be expected when such patients are treated. A meta-analysis of 123 randomized trials of drug treatment in elderly patients demonstrated that to prevent one stroke, 22 patients needed to be treated for 5 years; the corresponding number for coronary heart disease is 45. These numbers are between 2 and 4 times lower than the equivalent number needed to treat in younger adults.

2.1.2 Smoking

Cigarette smoking increases the risk of myocardial infarction, stroke and peripheral vascular disease and cessation for as little as 1 to 5 years markedly reduces the risk. There is no evidence that the benefits are any less with age.

2.1.3 Hypercholesterolaemia

In the age group 65–74 years, 38% of men and 68% of women have a plasma total cholesterol level of 6.5 mmol/l or above. However, the key coronary heart disease prevention trials had an upper age limit of 70 (Scandinavian Simvastatin Survival Study) and 64 (West of Scotland Coronary Prevention Study) respectively. The recent Standing Medical Advisory Committee guidelines recommend prescribing 3-hydroxy-3-methylglutaryl coenzyme A (HMG CoA) reductase inhibitors ('statins') to patients who have had a myocardial infarction with a total cholesterol of 4.8 mmol/l or more and those with angina or other atherosclerotic disease (including stroke or peripheral vascular disease) with a total cholesterol of 5.5 mmol/l or more. There is no guidance on secondary prevention in those over 70 and considerable concerns have been raised about the cost-effectiveness of this approach, even in those under 70. A similar issue is raised with primary prevention, where statins are recommended for patients less than 70 years with a cholesterol level of 5.5 mmol/l or more and a high risk of developing coronary heart disease. It is not clear whether this strategy should also be applied to patients over 70.

2.1.4 Other Risk Factors

Diabetes is a greater risk factor for elderly women who are twice as likely as men to develop non-insulin-dependent diabetes. Physical inactivity is an independent risk factor and moderate exercise reduces coronary risk, even in older age groups. Excess alcohol leads to an increased risk of haemorrhagic stroke and recommended limits should be adhered to (i.e. 14–21 units/week for women, 21–28 units/week for men). Following myocardial infarction proven effective secondary preventive measures include aspirin, beta-blockers and angiotensin-converting enzyme inhibitors (in patients with left ventricular dysfunction). None of these interventions should be denied on the basis of age alone.

2.2 HYPERTENSION IN OLD AGE

In industrialized societies, both systolic and diastolic BP tend to rise until the age of 60. After that, systolic pressure may continue to rise but diastolic pressure tends to stabilize or decline. In those under 80 years of age, treatment is recommended for mixed hypertension (systolic BP >160 mmHg, diastolic BP >90 mmHg) or for isolated systolic hypertension (systolic BP >160 mmHg, diastolic BP <90 mmHg), having ensured that the BP is persistently elevated on at least three occasions. In the biologically young over 80, the same guidelines apply.

2.2.1 Aetiology

Primary hypertension is responsible for 90% of cases. Secondary causes are no different than in younger patients but medication including over-the-counter drugs may be particularly relevant in elderly patients (Table 2.1). Renovascular hypertension increases with age to become the main cause of secondary hypertension in this age group.

2.2.2 Signs and Symptoms

Hypertension is usually a silent disease unless there is target organ involvement or secondary hypertension. Phaeochromocytoma may be associated with headache, flushing and blood pressure lability. Occlusive renal arterial disease may produce a sudden worsening of hypertension, with hypertensive heart failure, headaches and renal artery bruits which are particularly significant if they occur in diastole. Patients with renal parenchymal disease may experience recurrent urinary tract infection, frequency, nocturia, haematuria and anaemia. Thyroid disease should be considered in elderly patients with recent onset hypertension without renal or other cause. Patients with Conn's syndrome exhibit muscle weakness, nocturia and hypokalaemic alkalosis. Cushing's disease is suggested by hypokalaemic alkalosis and a typical physical appearance.

Table 2.1   Principal causes of secondary hypertension in old age

---

Underlying diseases
Renovascular disease
Renal parenchymal diseases (e.g. diabetic nephropathy)
Cushing's disease and syndrome
Primary hyperaldosteronism
Phaeochromocytoma
Hypercalcaemia
Thyroid disease

Drugs and chemicals
Non-steroidal anti-inflammatory drugs
Monoamine oxidase inhibitors (MAOIs)
Corticosteroids
Oestrogens
Beta-adrenergic receptor agonists
Excess alcohol
Excess salt

2.2.3   Diagnosis

The diagnosis of hypertension depends on finding elevated arterial pressure on at least three separate occasions with at least two BP measurements on each occasion. The technique of ambulatory blood pressure measurement is useful when 'white coat' hypertension is suspected or for the diagnosis of isolated systolic hypertension. It is also useful to assess nocturnal 'dipper status' and blood pressure variability over 24 hours. Patients who do not 'dip' at night to give lower BP readings or those who have a great deal of variability in the readings throughout the 24 hours are more likely to develop cardiovascular complications. The phenomenon of 'pseudohypertension' is sometimes seen in older hypertensives. This refers to overestimation of (usually systolic) blood pressure in the absence of signs of end organ damage. Osler's sign is said to indicate the presence of pseudohypertension, in which the brachial or radial artery remains palpable after the blood pressure cuff is inflated to suprasystolic levels, although the accuracy of this sign in predicting pseudohypertension is unknown.

Baseline investigation includes serum, urea, electrolytes, calcium, glucose and cholesterol, full blood count, thyroid function (if indicated)

and urinalysis. Electrocardiography should be performed to look for left ventricular hypertrophy with or without strain pattern. Echocardiography is not routinely indicated but may help if the BP is borderline and more definitive evidence of left ventricular hypertrophy is needed before deciding to treat.

2.2.4   Treatment

Non-pharmacological Treatment

Non-pharmacological measures include maintaining an ideal body weight, avoiding excessive alcohol intake, controlling dietary sodium, exercising regularly and avoiding smoking. These measures may lower BP in some patients and allow a reduction in the number and doses of antihypertensives in others.

Pharmacological Treatment

The current guidelines from the British Hypertension Society recommended diuretics or beta-blockers as first-line agents, with angiotensin-converting enzyme (ACE) inhibitors, calcium channel blockers and alpha-blockers to be used when the first two are contraindicated or ineffective. The role of these newer agents as first-line agents continues to be debated because most of them have not been evaluated in long-term outcome trials. The recent Syst-Eur trial evaluated the treatment of isolated systolic hypertension in the elderly with the dihydropyridine calcium channel blocker nitrendipine with the addition of the ACE inhibitor enalapril and the thiazide diuretic hydrochlorothiazide if necessary. A reduction in stroke and other cardiovascular complications was demonstrated and the benefit occurred soon after randomization when most patients were still on monotherapy with nitrendipine. First-line treatment with long-acting calcium antagonists (and possibly ACE inhibitors) can therefore be recommended in the elderly, if thiazides and beta-blockers are unsuitable.

When starting treatment (Table 2.2), the lowest recommended dose should be chosen. If it is partially effective the dose should be increased except in the case of the thiazides. If this is not completely effective another drug should be added, preferably one with a complementary

Table 2.2 Agents which may be used in hypertension

Drug class	Adverse effects	Comments
Thiazides	Hypokalaemia Hyponatraemia Hypomagnesaemia Decreased glucose tolerance Increased serum urate Increased creatinine Increased LDL Impotence	May aggravate diabetes or gout Low doses as effective as higher with fewer adverse effects Ineffective in severe renal failure Indapamide may be used in diabetes
Beta-blockers	Fatigue Depression Sleep disturbance	Lipophilic beta-blockers more likely to cause central effects (e.g. metoprolol) Contraindicated in asthma, CCF, PVD, IDDM Relatively less effective in elderly Water soluble agents accumulate in renal failure—reduce dose
Calcium antagonists	Headache Flushing Constipation Ankle oedema	Adverse effects less with newer agents (e.g. amlodipine—except at higher dose) Safe in diabetes, COPD, PVD Useful in combination with ACE inhibitors Avoid short-acting dihydropyridines
ACE inhibitors	Cough Hyperkalaemia Renal failure	Renal failure may be precipitated if patient on NSAIDs or has bilateral renal artery stenosis Avoid potassium-sparing diuretics Safe in diabetes
Alpha-blockers	Postural hypotension	Much less with doxazosin Favourable effects on lipids Safe in diabetes and renal failure
Angiotensin-II antagonists	Hyperkalaemia Renal failure	Very well tolerated Caution if renal artery stenosis suspected Avoid potassium-sparing diuretics Monitor renal function Safe in diabetes
Moxonidine	Sedation Dry mouth Nausea Dizziness	Well tolerated May be indicated in patients who have adverse effects with other drugs Avoid in Raynaud's, PVD, conduction defects, unstable angina, CCF Reduce dose in renal failure Safe in diabetes

LDL, low density lipoprotein; CCF, congestive cardiac failure; PVD, peripheral vascular disease; IDDM, insulin-dependent diabetes mellitus; COPD, chronic obstructive pulmonary disease.

action to the first drug (e.g. thiazides and ACE inhibitors). If the patient develops side-effects the drug should be stopped or the dose reduced (e.g. swollen ankles with calcium channel blockers).

There have been some recent misgivings about the long-term safety of calcium antagonists, following reports in 1995 suggesting significantly increased cardiovascular mortality in patients receiving short-acting nifedipine as an antihypertensive agent. In 1996, a further report suggested that individuals taking long-term calcium antagonists had a significantly higher incidence of cancer. Although the methodologies and interpretations of these reports have been criticized and a clear cause and effect relationship between calcium antagonist therapy and these adverse outcomes has not been established, uncertainty regarding the long-term safety of shorter-acting calcium antagonists in particular remains and will persist until further studies refute or confirm these findings.

2.3 ISCHAEMIC HEART DISEASE IN OLD AGE

Coronary artery disease is not only more common in elderly people but also more severe, with a greater incidence of left main stem and three vessel disease. The diagnosis of angina can usually be made from the history without further investigations. However, if the history is atypical, or symptoms are poorly controlled or it is thought that prognosis should be more precisely established, exercise tolerance testing may help, although lack of fitness or coexistent neurological, peripheral vascular or musculoskeletal disease may make it difficult to perform in this age group. If exercise testing is not feasible or appropriate, a myocardial perfusion scan with intravenous adenosine infusion (to produce vaso-dilatation and reflex tachycardia) may help to demonstrate revers-ible ischaemia.

2.3.1 Medical Therapy of Angina

Aspirin
The routine use of aspirin 75–300 mg in patients with chronic stable angina reduces the incidence of non-fatal myocardial infarction. Gastro-

intestinal side-effects may be reduced by using lower doses but not by the use of enteric coated preparations.

Nitrates

Sublingual or buccal nitrates in tablet or spray form may be taken to relieve discomfort or before precipitating activities. Headache or light-headedness may be ameliorated if the patient sits. If glyceryl trinitrate (GTN) tablets are used the supply must be renewed every 6 weeks, beyond which tablets deteriorate.

Prophylactic Treatment

Frail patients or those with very occasional symptoms may be managed with GTN and aspirin alone but all others should have treatment with a prophylactic anti-anginal such as a beta-blocker, calcium antagonist or long-acting nitrate. The efficacy of nitrates is variable and may decrease after 4–6 weeks of treatment because of the development of nitrate tolerance. A 'nitrate-free' period is recommended by using modified-release once daily preparations (e.g. isosorbide mononitrate 60–120 mg o.d.) or a short-acting preparation twice a day. Beta-blockers are very effective but are contraindicated in the presence of asthma, chronic obstructive pulmonary disease, peripheral vascular disease, heart failure or atrioventricular (AV) nodal disease. A cardioselective beta-blocker such as metoprolol or atenolol should be used, but tiredness or cold extremities may be disabling for some elderly patients. If symptoms continue, a calcium antagonist or nitrate should be added. The combination of a beta-blocker with verapamil or diltiazem can cause symptomatic bradycardia or AV block, and amlodipine or a long-acting form of nifedipine is preferred. All calcium antagonists can cause hypotension and flushing, nifedipine and amlodipine can cause ankle oedema, and constipation may be a particular problem with verapamil. If the patient has impaired left ventricular function, diltiazem and verapamil should be avoided because of their greater negative inotropic effects.

Nicorandil activates ATP-dependent potassium channels thereby increasing the entry of potassium ions into vascular smooth muscle cells, which results in smooth muscle relaxation. It also increases potassium influx into ischaemic cardiac myocytes and reduces their contractile activity. In clinical studies, the anti-anginal efficacy of nicorandil was found to be similar to that of atenolol and diltiazem. The only frequent adverse effect is headache, which tends to diminish with frequent use. Other adverse effects include dizziness, hypotension, palpitation and gastrointestinal disorders. It is contraindicated in left ventricular failure with low pressures because it reduces both preload and afterload. Its place in therapy is currently uncertain but it may be used if other agents are contraindicated or as an add-on agent with conventional regimens.

2.3.2 Interventional Treatment for Angina

Most elderly people obtain adequate symptom control from anti-anginal treatment. Coronary angioplasty or bypass grafting should be reserved for those who do not respond to medication. Coronary arteriography will demonstrate the extent and severity of coronary artery disease and degree of left ventricular dysfunction, which are the main determinants of a patient's suitability for intervention.

Percutaneous transluminal coronary angioplasty (PTCA) can offer better symptomatic relief than medical therapy in patients with single vessel disease but there is a significant risk of complications. Initial success rates for PTCA in elderly patients are in the order of 84–96%, with major complication rates of 3–6%. Long-term event-free survival is 68–76%, and probably relates to left ventricular function, progression of the coronary disease and development of non-cardiac disease. There is also a role for angioplasty of a single 'culprit lesion' in patients with multi-vessel diseases.

The mortality figures for **coronary artery bypass grafting (CABG)** in the elderly range from 2 to 10% and depend on whether patients smoke, are very elderly (>75 years) or have impaired left ventricular function. About 75% of patients are rendered angina-free at long-term follow-up.

2.3.3 Unstable Angina

The management of unstable angina should differ little from that of younger patients and should initially include bed rest, aspirin, beta-blockers, nitrates and heparin. If the pain is not satisfactorily controlled then coronary arteriography is indicated in this age group as in younger patients. Angioplasty of CABG may then be performed as indicated.

2.3.4   Myocardial Infarction

Modern management of myocardial infarction now includes thrombolysis to limit myocardial damage, improve left ventricular function and reduce mortality. Despite evidence from the major trials such as GISSI, ISIS-2 and GUSTO that thrombolysis is as effective in the elderly as in the young and results in a greater absolute reduction in mortality, only a small proportion of this age group receive it. This is partly because older patients present later and the typical features of infarction (such as pain) may be absent. However, in addition, many doctors are reluctant to consider thrombolytic therapy in the elderly because they wrongly assume that old age is a contraindication. Thrombolytic therapy should not be withheld on the basis of age alone.

2.4   HEART FAILURE

The prevalence of heart failure has increased in the elderly in recent years as the general population has aged and survival rates following myocardial infarction have improved. The symptoms of fatigue, shortness of breath and oedema are due to inadequate perfusion of tissues during exertion in association with fluid retention. Coronary artery disease, hypertension and valvular disorders are the commonest causes of systolic dysfunction in the elderly although a history of angina and myocardial infarction may be absent in many. Hypertrophic, dilated cardiomyopathy (idiopathic or due to alcohol) or restrictive cardiomyopathy due to amyloid may be also seen in this age group. Rarely, mitral valve prolapse may present with heart failure.

Regardless of the underlying aetiology, the symptoms of heart failure may be precipitated by non-compliance with drug or dietary regimens including a low salt diet, use of non-steroidal anti-inflammatory drugs (NSAIDs), onset of atrial fibrillation or myocardial infarction. Systemic precipitants include anaemia, chest infection and thyrotoxicosis. The diagnosis may be more difficult in the elderly in whom an unrelated dementia or confusion may limit the examiner's ability to obtain a reliable history. Physical findings may also be difficult to interpret but a gallop rhythm is a reliable indicator of left ventricular overload even in elderly patients. An electrocardiogram (ECG) will define cardiac rhythm and provides evidence of previous infarction or left ventricular hypertrophy. Chest radiography should be performed to look for pulmonary congestion and effusions. Echocardiography is usually indicated to delineate the presence and extent of wall motion abnormalities and the severity of ventricular dysfunction. An ejection fraction of less than 45% is evidence of left ventricular dysfunction. Other abnormalities may be detected such as diastolic left ventricular dysfunction (particularly important in the elderly), left ventricular hypertrophy, valvular lesions and pericardial effusion. Full blood count, renal and thyroid function tests are also helpful to detect compounding abnormalities such as polycythaemia, renal impairment and hypo/hyperthyroidism.

2.4.1 Treatment of Acute Left Ventricular Failure

Acute left ventricular failure is usually produced by redistribution of blood from vasoconstricted peripheral vascular beds to the central compartment. An intravenous loop diuretic such as frusemide (see below) should be given with an opiate and oxygen. The rapid effectiveness of frusemide is due to its early venodilator effect which encourages peripheral venous pooling rather than to its diuretic or natriuretic effects, which occur later. Sublingual or intravenous glyceryl trinitrate may be useful in reducing cardiac preload.

2.4.2 Treatment of Chronic Congestive Cardiac Failure

Treatment is aimed at relieving symptoms and delaying the progression of left ventricular dysfunction.

Non-pharmacological Management
Salt restriction to 2 to 3 g per day will reduce a patient's need for diuretic therapy and regular non-isometric exercise will increase peak exercise capacity. Patients should limit their consumption of alcohol to 2 units per day and refrain completely if they have alcoholic cardiomyopathy.

Diuretics

Diuretics relieve pulmonary and peripheral oedema. Thiazide diuretics administered two to three times weekly may be adequate to maintain normal intravascular volume in mild congestive heart failure but the daily administration of a loop diuretic such as frusemide or bumetanide is necessary when the congestion is more severe or when impaired renal function reduces the responsiveness to thiazides. Diuretics should be slowly titrated starting with the lowest effective dose, depending on the severity of the congestive heart failure at presentation. Response to therapy is assessed by measuring the central venous pressure. Elevated pressure in the internal jugular vein or the presence of hepatojugular reflux suggests the need for more aggressive therapy unless the patient has symptomatic hypotension or a progressively rising urea concentration or tricuspid regurgitation.

A once-daily dose of a loop diuretic is usually sufficient but those with more persistent fluid retention may require two doses per day. In severe cases admission to hospital for several days of intravenous frusemide is useful. This is because the absorption of frusemide, which is erratic under normal circumstances, may become even less predictable in congestive heart failure due to small intestinal mucosal oedema. An alternative strategy is to switch to oral bumetanide. When venous pressure remains high the administration of a thiazide (e.g. bendrofluazide 2.5 mg) or metolazone (2.5–5 mg), which have a different site of action in the renal tubule, may be effective. Thiazide and loop diuretics share similar adverse effects of hypovolaemia, hyponatraemia, hypomagnesaemia, azotaemia, hyperglycaemia and hyperuricaemia. The age-associated reductions in renal function and dietary and fluid intake increase the risks of these problems in the elderly. Regular measurements of serum potassium, sodium and renal function are necessary during diuretic therapy and development of fatigue, hypotension or progressively raised urea calls for a dose reduction and temporary cessation of therapy. An increased intake of potassium usually in the form of potassium supplements or a potassium-sparing diuretic (e.g. amiloride 5 mg) may be needed to keep the potassium concentration above 4 mmol/l.

Angiotensin-converting Enzyme Inhibitors

The most significant pharmacological advance in the treatment of heart failure in the past two decades has been the introduction of ACE inhibitors. These agents have been consistently shown to improve the survival of patients with chronic heart failure. They also prevent heart failure and reduce mortality in patients who have had a myocardial infarction associated with signs or symptoms of acute heart failure or a reduction in ejection fraction. Therapy should be initiated in a low dose (e.g. 12.5 mg captopril twice a day or 2.5 mg enalapril once a day) in patients with heart failure and the first dose (captopril 6.25 mg) given under supervision. Even lower doses should be given if the patient's serum sodium is less than 135 mmol/l, which indicates a high level of renin activity. Although these agents are generally well tolerated in the elderly, symptomatic hypotension, progressive rise in urea and creatinine concentrations or an intractable, non-productive cough may necessitate reducing or stopping the ACE inhibitor. These agents tend to conserve potassium by reducing the secretion of aldosterone, so patients on diuretics generally do not need supplemental potassium or a potassium-sparing diuretic. Preliminary evidence suggests that the angiotensin-II receptor blockers such as losartan may be better tolerated and result in a better survival rate than ACE inhibitors in elderly patients with heart failure.

Other Vasodilators

The combination of hydralazine and isosorbide dinitrate has been demonstrated to improve survival in clinical trials involving patients with congestive heart failure who were also given digoxin and diuretics. The effect on survival was not as favourable as with enalapril, however. They should be considered for patients who cannot tolerate ACE inhibitors or who remain symptomatic while taking an ACE inhibitor, although no trials with the second group have been performed. The dose of these vasodilators needs to be individualized and poor tolerance limits their usefulness.

Digoxin

The therapeutic efficacy of digoxin in patients with heart failure and normal sinus rhythm has long been debated. A recently completed trial (the Digitalis Investigation Group (DIG) study), noted no significant effect of digoxin on mortality but a reduction in the hospitalization rate for heart failure compared with placebo. Patients with heart failure who have not responded well to diuretics and vasodilators may therefore benefit from digoxin as well as those patients who are in atrial fibrillation.

Beta-blockers

Treatment with beta-blockers such as carvedilol or metoprolol may have the potential to reduce morbidity and mortality in heart failure but there is no unequivocal evidence as yet.

Anticoagulant Therapy

Patients with heart failure who are at particularly high risk of thrombo-embolism, e.g. those with a history of thromboembolism or those with atrial fibrillation, should receive maintenance anticoagulation.

Surgical Treatment

Although drugs are the mainstay of treatment for heart failure, surgery does have an important place. Coronary artery revascularization may occasionally improve left ventricular function dramatically by improving myocardial blood flow provided that there is sufficient viable 'hibernat-ing' myocardium. Finally, cardiac transplantation is now being performed in patients up to 70 years with good results.

2.5 CARDIAC REHABILITATION IN OLD AGE

Cardiac rehabilitation may be useful for some patients who have suffered a myocardial infarction and some who have severe heart failure. The goal is to help the patient maintain or regain his/her independence. Each patient responds differently to the stress of severe illness so the programme must be individualized. Typically the patient begins with light activity and progresses to moderate activity under the guidance of a physiotherapist or nurse. Following a myocardial infarction, activity should be minimized initially but then gradually increased. On the other hand, patients with unstable angina should not be exercised at all and patients with severe heart failure should only be exercised under the supervision of a trained attendant in a well equipped cardiac rehabilita-tion facility. When they are discharged home patients should be given a detailed home activity programme. Ongoing support is necessary during this emotionally stressful period. It must be made clear to the patients which activities can be undertaken and which should be avoided. Although elderly patients may not ask about resuming sexual activity they can be advised that it is safe to do so but that they should avoid over-exertion and rest as necessary.

2.6 ATRIAL FIBRILLATION IN OLD AGE

The prevalence of atrial fibrillation increases with age and affects 2–4% of individuals over 60 and 11.6% of those over 75 years. It is associated with rheumatic heart disease (particularly mitral valve disease), ischaemic heart disease, hypertension, thyrotoxicosis, increased alcohol consumption and bronchopulmonary disease. Paroxysmal atrial fibrillation may occur in sick sinus syndrome. In about 30% of cases no underlying aetiology is found and the term 'lone atrial fibrillation' is used. Patients with newly diagnosed atrial fibrillation should have an ECG, chest X-ray, echocardiogram, thyroid function tests, renal function and electrolytes.

2.6.1 Treatment

The goals of treatment are to minimize symptoms and decrease the incidence of complications.

Acute Onset of Atrial Fibrillation
There is a high rate of cardioversion when the atrial fibrillation is of short duration (less than 48 hours). Patients who are clinically stable can be observed for a few hours. If spontaneous cardioversion fails to occur this can be attempted chemically or electrically. Flecainide 2 mg/kg given intravenously over 10 to 30 minutes cardioverts up to 90% of cases. It has significant negative inotropic and proarrhythmic effects and should be avoided in patients with severely impaired left ventricular function and coronary artery disease. Serum potassium should be within the normal range and resuscitation equipment available. Anticoagulation is not needed before electrical cardioversion if the atrial fibrillation is of

less than 48 hours' duration since there is insufficient time for thrombus to form within the fibrillating atria. It the patient is haemodynamically compromised, he/she should immediately be cardioverted or treated with rate-limiting therapy.

Chronic Atrial Fibrillation

Digoxin is the most frequently used agent to control heart rate in a trial fibrillation. It acts by enhancing vagal tone at the AV node. Its mechanism of action means that it provides poor rate control in situations of increased sympathetic output such as during exercise. The addition of beta-blockers, verapamil or diltiazem can normalize heart rate response. If verapamil is chosen the dose of digoxin may need to be reduced since verapamil increases serum digoxin levels. When rapid control is needed (e.g. when the atrial fibrillation has precipitated left ventricular failure) intravenous amiodarone is the drug of choice.

Cardioversion to sinus rhythm should be attempted once in most patients with chronic atrial fibrillation except those with severe mitral valve disease and a markedly dilated left atrium in whom it is generally not successful. Patients need to be fully anticoagulated and although sinus rhythm is achieved in about 85% of cases, recurrence of a trial fibrillation is common. This is less likely to occur if the patient is maintained on sotalol but its proarrhythmic potential in patients with left ventricular dysfunction, previous ventricular arrhythmia, bradycardia or a long QT interval means that it is contraindicated in many patients. The alternative is amiodarone, which is very effective but may be associated with significant adverse effects such as pulmonary fibrosis, thyroid dysfunction or photosensitivity in some patients.

Antithrombotic Treatment of Atrial Fibrillation

In atrial fibrillation the disturbance in blood flow predisposes to the formation of atrial thrombi. Up to 20% of patients with acute stroke present with atrial fibrillation. The risk of thromboembolism is particularly high in patients with rheumatic heart disease who should always be anticoagulated with warfarin. Most elderly patients with non-rheumatic atrial fibrillation should be anticoagulated with warfarin or aspirin unless there are clear contraindications. Several large clinical trials have demonstrated a reduction in embolic phenomena of about 65% at international normalized ratios (INRs) between 1.5 and 4.5 in patients treated with warfarin. On the other hand, aspirin is simpler to monitor and carries a lower risk of bleeding although it is less effective than warfarin in primary and secondary prevention of stroke. Before starting treatment with warfarin or aspirin it is important to balance the risks (especially bleeding) and benefits in a particular patient (Table 2.3). Echocardiography may help with risk stratification in that a large left atrium, impaired left ventricular function or intracardiac thrombus are all associated with an increased risk of thromboembolism. To minimize the risk of intracranial bleeding with prophylactic warfarin, hypertension should be adequately controlled and the risks and benefits of anti-coagulation reviewed annually. Factors that may increase the risk of bleeding with warfarin are listed in Table 2.4.

The risk of bleeding in patients taking oral anticoagulants increases as the INR increases. The recommended target INR in patients with atrial fibrillation is 2.0–3.0 except for patients with mechanical prosthetic heart valves or previous thromboembolic stroke in whom a ratio of 3.0–4.5 should be maintained. Patients should be reviewed regularly at anticoagulation clinics to optimize control and should be educated about drug interaction and the risk of bleeding.

Table 2.3   Risk stratification and selection of prophylaxis in non-rheumatic atrial fibrillation

---

High risk of stroke—warfarin unless contraindicated
Previous transient ischaemic attack or stroke,
   age over 75 with diabetes
   and/or hypertension

Moderate risk—aspirin as effective as warfarin
Age <65 with diabetes
   and/or hypertension
Age 65–74 with or without diabetes
   and/or hypertension
Age >75

Low risk—aspirin
Age <65
   normal left ventricular function, atrial size on echocardiography
   no hypertension or diabetes

Table 2.4   Factors that may increase the risk of bleeding from warfarin

Advanced age
Frequent falls
Uncontrolled hypertension (systolic BP >180 mmHg; diastolic BP >100 mmHg
Alcohol excess
Liver disease
Poor compliance
Gastrointestinal blood loss
Previous cerebral haemorrhage
Coagulation defects, thrombocytopenia
Concomitant use of aspirin

2.7 VALVULAR HEART DISEASE

Valvular disorders in old age result from rheumatic endocarditis in
earlier life or predominantly from age-related degeneration. The decline
in rheumatic fever and the increased longevity of the population have
changed the prevalence and character of valvular heart disease: mitral
stenosis and rheumatic aortic stenosis are seen less frequently. Stenosis
caused by degeneration in congenitally bicuspid or previously normal
valves is the commonest cause of aortic stenosis and the ageing mitral
valve may become regurgitant if heavily calcified. The improvement in
outcome from cardiac surgery means that elderly people with valve
disease should be assessed carefully for valve replacement if surgery is
indicated.

2.7.1 Aortic Stenosis

Severe, symptomatic aortic stenosis carries a high mortality if left
untreated and one year survival may be as low as 57%. Aortic stenosis
presents with syncope, angina pectoris or heart failure. It is often
dismissed as aortic sclerosis or missed altogether in elderly patients in
whom the clinical signs are often less characteristic. Chest X-ray may
show an enlarged heart with calcium deposits in the valve and ECG will
show left ventricular hypertrophy with repolarization changes. Echocardiography will confirm the diagnosis and Doppler studies will give an
assessment of the pressure gradient across the valve. The major purpose

of cardiac catheterization is to determine the presence and extent of coronary artery disease.

Management

The management of patients with asymptomatic severe aortic stenosis is controversial. Surgery is often indicated, especially if the aortic valve gradient is high (100 mmHg), or if the patient is particularly active. The development of dyspnoea on exertion, angina or syncope indicates an urgent need to replace the valve. The presence of left ventricular impairment due to aortic stenosis, however severe, is not a contra-indication to surgery. Aortic stenosis is curable by valve replacement, even in octogenarians, although the perioperative mortality rate is up to 15% in this age group. Patients requiring CABG in addition to valve replacement have poorer outcomes, with mortality rates of up to 20%.

2.7.2 Aortic Regurgitation

Isolated aortic regurgitation is uncommon in old age and usually occurs in association with aortic stenosis. Rare causes include dilatation of the aortic root in hypertension or chronic aortitis due to rheumatoid disease, Reiter's syndrome or syphilis. Acute aortic regurgitation is usually due to endocarditis or aortic dissection. Chronic aortic regurgitation has a long asymptomatic period and then presents with exertional dyspnoea, orthopnoea, paroxysmal nocturnal dyspnoea and palpitations. The ECG shows left ventricular hypertrophy and strain and the chest X-ray shows cardiomegaly in decompensated aortic regurgitation. Echocardiography demonstrates increased end-diastolic and end-systolic volumes and grades the severity of the aortic regurgitation. The regurgitation of radiocontrast from the aortic root into the left ventricle is demonstrated at catheterization.

Management

Chronic aortic regurgitation has a favourable prognosis, with 75% of patients surviving 5 years after diagnosis. The onset of symptoms heralds rapid deterioration. Patients who have no symptoms should be reviewed at 6-monthly intervals and left ventricular size and function assessed by echocardiography. Evidence of left ventricular dilatation, even in the absence of major symptoms, means that the patient should be considered for surgery, which is usually aortic valve replacement.

2.7.3 Mitral Stenosis

Rheumatic heart disease is the commonest cause of mitral stenosis although valve leaflet distortion from lupus endocarditis, amyloid infiltration and calcification can occasionally occur. Elderly patients with mitral stenosis tend to fall into two groups: those who have had mitral valvotomy previously for rheumatic disease and those with mild diseases who have only become symptomatic in later life. Patients present with dyspnoea and fatigue which may be gradual in onset. Haemoptysis due to pulmonary venous hypertension is uncommon in the elderly. Electrocardiogram usually shows atrial fibrillation and chest X-ray shows left atrial enlargement. Echocardiography can assess the severity of stenosis and the pulmonary artery pressure when tricuspid regurgitation is present. Elderly patients should have coronary angiography to look for concurrent coronary diseases.

Management
Most elderly people's symptoms can be improved by control of the atrial fibrillation with digoxin. Anticoagulation is recommended for all patients with mitral stenosis and is mandatory for patients in atrial fibrillation. Loop diuretics should be used to control pulmonary congestion. If symptoms are not relieved by medical therapy, patients should be considered for percutaneous balloon mitral valvuloplasty which is the treatment of choice if the valve is suitable (i.e. minimal or no calcification). Contraindications to the procedure include the presence of left atrial thrombus, severe subvalvar involvement or valve calcification and significant mitral regurgitation. The surgical alternatives are open mitral commissurotomy or mitral valve replacement. Mitral valve replacement carries a mortality of about 20% in the elderly.

2.7.4   Mitral Regurgitation

Rheumatic heart disease, myxomatous degeneration, ischaemia, prolapse or dilated cardiomyopathy may all lead to primary mitral valve regurgitation. Acute mitral regurgitation may occur if endocarditis destroys the leaflets or chordae and following myocardial infarction if there is sudden rupture of a papillary muscle. Chronic mitral regurgitation presents with fatigue and gradually decreasing exercise tolerance. Symptoms become troublesome when the ventricle starts to fail and the patient develops pulmonary vascular congestion. The ECG shows left atrial enlargement with P mitrale or atrial fibrillation. Chest X-ray shows left ventricular enlargement and sometimes calcification of the mitral valve with a lateral view. Echocardiography demonstrates left atrial and left ventricular function and dimensions, as well as the anatomy of the mitral valve. If surgery is being considered, transoesophageal echocardiography is needed to determine the suitability of the valve for repair.

Management

Symptoms may initially be controlled by diuretics, digoxin and ACE inhibitors but their onset indicates decompensation. Surgery improves survival in patients with symptomatic mitral regurgitation and both symptoms and left ventricular dilatation are indications for considering surgery. Surgical outcome is related to left ventricular function. When ejection fraction is <35% the risk of surgery is high at any age. The choice between mitral valve repair or replacement depends on the anatomy of the valve and the experience of the surgeon. Valve repair with preservation of the subvalvular apparatus appears to carry a lower risk and a better long-term prognosis for left ventricular function, embolism and infection.

2.8   INFECTIVE ENDOCARDITIS

More than half of all cases of infective endocarditis occur in patients over 60 years. About 40% of elderly people with endocarditis have either no valvular disease or previously undiagnosed disease. Of the 60% who do have valvular lesions, about 30% have rheumatic lesions, 25% calcified valves and 5% mitral valve prolapse.

2.8.1 Aetiology

The development of infective endocarditis involves the formation of thrombus in an area of increased turbulence followed by transient bacteraemia which allows the thrombus to be colonized. The source of bacteraemia may include the oral cavity, genitourinary (GU) tract (particularly after instrumentation), the gastrointestinal (GI) tract, skin, decubitus ulcers, surgical wounds and intravenous cannulae. *Streptococcus* species, usually from the mouth, account for 25–70% of endocarditis cases, although *S. viridans* is less common than in younger people. Enterococci, which often inhabit the GU and lower GI tracts, account for up to 25% of cases in elderly men, particularly if prostatic disease leads to recurrent urinary tract infection and instrumentation. *S. bovis* can be isolated in >25% of cases of endocarditis in patients over 55 years. Many of these cases are associated with underlying asymptomatic GI malignancies, especially of the colon. *Staphylococcus* species account for about 20–30% of endocarditis cases in the elderly. *S. aureus* endocarditis is often discovered incidentally at autopsy. *S. epidermidis* is the most frequent isolate in prosthetic valve endocarditis. Other rare causes include *Bacteroides* or *Candida*. Culture-negative endocarditis accounts for about 10–20% of cases and is usually due to prior antibiotic administration. Fastidious organisms, inadequate laboratory techniques, right-sided endocarditis or uraemia are other causes.

2.8.2 Signs and Symptoms

Fever is the commonest presenting feature of endocarditis. However, the presentation is often atypical in the elderly, with non-specific complaints of anorexia, fatigue, confusion and weight loss, so the diagnosis may be missed. Cardiac murmurs are found in >90% of patients due to predisposing valvular lesions or the infective process itself. Heart failure and splenomegaly may also be present. About 50% of patients will have peripheral manifestations such as petechiae, splinter haemorrhages,

Osler's nodes, Janeway lesions and Roth spots. Thromboemboli may involve the spleen or kidney. Patients with tricuspid endocarditis may present with pulmonary emboli and abscesses. Cerebral embolism and rupture of an intracranial mycotic aneurysm may present with cerebral haemorrhage.

2.8.3 Diagnosis

Positive blood cultures are the most important aid to diagnosis. Other features include a normochromic normocytic anaemia, raised erythrocyte sedimentation rate and C-reactive protein, proteinuria and haematuria. Echocardiography may detect valvular vegetations, valvular destruction and regurgitation. Transoesophageal echocardiography is more sensitive for detecting vegetations and is particularly useful when imaging by standard echocardiography is negative or difficult but the index of suspicion is high.

2.8.4 Treatment

In acutely ill patients treatment should be started immediately after obtaining blood cultures (× 4) and is based on the likely infective organism in the specific clinical setting (Table 2.5). Once the infecting organism is isolated from blood cultures the regimen should be altered if necessary. All cases should be treated in close liaison with the microbiology department. Indications for surgery in patients with endocarditis include haemodynamic deterioration from valve dysfunction, fungal endocarditis, persistent infection, repeated relapses, recurrent emboli and an unstable infected postoperative prosthetic valve.

2.8.5 Prophylaxis

Antibiotic prophylaxis is indicated for elderly patients with valvular heart disease undergoing dental procedures or instrumentation of the GI or GU systems (Table 2.6).

Table 2.5 Treatment of infective endocarditis

Organism	Regimen
Unknown (natural valve)	IV benzylpenicillin 1.2 g × 6 hourly plus IV flucloxacillin 2 g × 6 hourly plus IV gentamicin (80 mg initially)
Streptococcus viridans	IV benzylpenicillin 1.2 g × 4 hourly × 2 weeks plus IV gentamicin (80 mg initially) × 2 weeks then amoxycillin 500 mg × 8 hourly × 2 weeks
Enterococci Other *Streptococcus* species (natural valve)	IV benzylpenicillin 1.2 g × 4 hourly × 4 weeks plus IV gentamicin (80 mg initially) × 4 weeks
Penicillin allergy	IV vancomycin (1 g initially) plus IV gentamicin (80 mg initially)
Staphylococcus aureus *Staphylococcus epidermidis*	Flucloxacillin 1 g × 6 hourly × 4 weeks plus IV gentamicin (80 mg initially) × 2 weeks
Penicillin allergy	IV vancomycin (1 g initially) × at least 4 weeks

Gentamicin and vancomycin levels are measured within 24 hours to determine subsequent doses.
IV, intravenous.

2.9 CARDIAC PACING

The NGB code is an international code to identify pacing systems. It consists of five letters and the first three identify the chamber being paced, the chamber being sensed and the sensing mode. Pacemakers with an ability to modify the pacing rate in response to exercise or emotion are referred to as 'rate responsive' or 'rate adaptive' systems and are identified by the fourth letter of the code. The fifth letter is rarely used and refers to the presence or absence of an anti-tachycardia function.

Pacing may be considered for one of two reasons: either for symptomatic benefit or to improve prognosis. The commonest syndromes to require pacing are sinus node disease, AV block, sinus node disease with AV block, atrial fibrillation with AV block and carotid and vasovagal syncope syndromes. Syncope or near-syncope are the most frequent

Table 2.6   Prophylaxis for infective endocarditis

Procedure	Regimen
Dental procedures (local anaesthesia)	Oral amoxycillin 3 g taken 1 hour before procedure
Penicillin allergy or >1 dose penicillin in previous month	Clindamycin 600 mg
Previous endocarditis	IV amoxicillin 1 g plus IV gentamicin 120 mg oral amoxycillin 500 mg 6 hours later
Dental procedures (general anaesthesia)	IV amoxicillin 1 g at induction then oral amoxycillin 500 mg 6 hours later add IV gentamicin 120 mg at induction for **high-risk*** patient
Penicillin allergy or >1 dose penicillin in previous month	IV vancomycin 1 g over 100 minutes then IV gentamicin 120 mg at induction
Upper respiratory tract procedures	As above: post-procedure dose given parenterally if swallowing painful
GU procedures	As for high-risk group above
GI procedures	As for high-risk group above but only patients with previous endocarditis or prosthetic valves

*High-risk patients have prosthetic valves or previous endocarditis.
IV, intravenous.

indications for pacing. Twenty-four hour Holter monitoring may show asymptomatic bradycardia or pauses. If these exceed three seconds in a patient with recurrent syncope, a pacemaker implantation should be considered. Intermittent second degree heart and complete AV block may be life-threatening and pacemaker implantation reduces the risk of sudden death. Although patients with carotid sinus and vagovagal syndromes (see Chapter 3) can vary greatly in their response to pacing, it is of most value where the predominant feature is bradycardia rather than vasodepression.

The selection of a pacemaker mode will depend on the condition but it is recommended that the ventricle should be paced if there is threatened or actual AV block and the atrium should be paced or sensed unless contraindicated. Patients with sinus node disease usually have intact AV conduction. Single chamber atrial adaptive rate pacing will reproduce many of the features of sinus rhythm, maintaining AV synchrony at all paced heart rates. If there is any doubt about the integrity of AV nodal function, a dual chamber system should be chosen. For patients with second or third degree AV block a dual chamber pacemaker is required to maintain atrial synchrony. Sinus node disease with AV block needs a dual chamber pacemaker with an added adaptive rate feature to overcome the AV block and to allow an increase in heart rate during exercise. Single chamber ventricular pacing with appropriate rate response is appropriate for patients with atrial fibrillation with AV block. Dual chamber pacing is required to correct the bradycardia of carotid sinus and vasovagal syndromes. Rate hysteresis will avoid pacing the physiological bradycardia which occurs during sleep but will allow immediate pacing of asystole. The majority of iatrogenic morbidity in cardiac pacing arises from the use of single chamber ventricular pacing in the presence of spontaneous atrial contraction against closed tricuspid and mitral valves ('pacemaker syndrome'). Acutely raised atrial pressure impedes venous return, leading to underfilling of the ventricles during the next diastolic period with resultant reduction in stroke volume. The result may be symptoms of hypotension and syncope or near-syncope, dizziness, dyspnoea and weakness, worse whilst standing. Atrioventricular (dual chamber) pacing or, when AV conduction is intact, atrial pacing will avoid these problems.

2.10　PERIPHERAL VASCULAR DISEASE

2.10.1　Intermittent Claudication

Intermittent claudication occurs with an estimated prevalence of 5% among people over 60. It is twice as common in men as in women and the risk factors are those of generalized atherosclerosis, with smoking and hypertension being thought to be particularly important. Intermittent claudication may be exacerbated by beta-blockers, particularly those with a vasodilator action such as pindolol, carvedilol and labetalol, although more conventional agents such as atenolol, metoprolol and propranolol may be well tolerated in patients with stable peripheral vascular disease. Claudication due to arterial disease must be distinguished from neurogenic and venous claudication as well as joint disease. Patients with mild arterial occlusion may have normal foot pulses at rest and measurement of brachial : ankle blood pressure ratio using hand-held Doppler devices may be very helpful for diagnosis, particularly where patients have obvious coexistent venous disease or arthritis. Magnetic resonance imaging is the investigation of choice for detecting neurogenic claudication. Three-quarters of patients with vascular claudication stabilize within a few months of onset of symptoms, and the prognosis is determined more by the high incidence of coexistent coronary and cerebrovascular disease. The 10-year survival of patients with vascular claudication is approximately 50%. The management of intermittent claudication is detailed in Table 2.7.

2.10.2 Acute Lower Limb Arterial Occlusion

The majority of patients presenting with acute lower limb ischaemia are elderly people with atrial fibrillation who are not treated with anticoagulants. Cardiogenic embolism may also result from recent transmural myocardial infarction, valvular heart disease, ventricular aneurysm, atrial myxoma and paradoxical embolism from a patent foramen ovale. Aorto-iliac embolism may originate from aneurysms, disseminated atherosclerosis and prosthetic grafts. Occasionally, widespread cholesterol embolism occurs following aortic plaque rupture, resulting in ischaemic digits, renal impairment and delirium. This disorder may be associated with a false positive, low-titre anti-neutrophilic cytoplasmic antibody (ANCA) test, leading to an incorrect diagnosis of acute vasculitis.

The classical symptoms of acute lower limb ischaemia are pain, pallor, 'polor' (coldness), pulselessness and paraesthesiae. However, in frail elderly people, the presentation may be one of delirium, 'off-legs' or 'taken-to-the-bed', which often leads to delayed diagnosis and a fatal outcome from acute renal failure (rhabdomyolysis) and gangrene. The diagnosis may then be easily missed unless skin temperature, peripheral pulses and lower limb colour are carefully noted. Since over 90% of cases are due to embolism, surgical consultation should be sought immediately with a view to emergency embolectomy. In the meantime, patients should be treated with intravenous heparin infusion. If embolectomy with a balloon catheter is not technically feasible or unsuccessful, an alternative is thrombolysis with intra-arterial infusion of tissue

Table 2.7   Management of intermittent claudication

(a) Non-pharmacological
    Stop smoking
    Regular exercise

(b) Pharmacological
    Low-dose aspirin
    Antihypertensive therapy as required
    Avoid vasodilators (e.g. pentoxifylline, naftidrofuryl, nicotinic acid derivatives
    etc.—tend to cause diversion of blood flow from ischaemic zone)

(c) Surgical
    Percutaneous transluminal angioplasty (± stenting) for iliac artery occlusion (75%
    patency rate at 5 years) for persistent, disabling claudication that does not
    respond to conservative therapy. PTA for stenoses below the inguinal ligament
    less effective: 40% patency rate at 5 years. Should only be done where there are
    facilities for management of acute arterial occlusion or rupture. May be done as
    day case procedure.
    Bypass surgery: results significantly better than PTA (5-year patency rate for
    iliac occlusions 95%, for femoropopliteal occlusions 70%)

plasminogen activator, streptokinase or urokinase. In situations where
intra-arterial access is not feasible, intravenous thrombolytic therapy
may be tried (as for acute myocardial infarction) but the outcome from
this form of therapy is much less certain.

All patients with cardiac emboli require anticoagulation with heparin
following reperfusion of the limb by embolectomy or thrombolysis. This
should then be followed by life-long anticoagulation with warfarin.

2.10.3   Rest Pain (Pre-Gangrene Ischaemia)

Lower limb ischaemic pain at rest usually signifies impending gangrene,
requires strong opiate analgesia with morphine or diamorphine and
urgent surgical consultation with a view to reperfusion with vascular
reconstruction if this is feasible or amputation if surgery is not feasible.
Conservative management may be necessary in some elderly patients
who are too frail for reconstructive or amputation surgery or if they
decline to have surgery. Sometimes, it may be possible to stabilize such
patients with such measures as:

- maintaining the limb in a dependent position (i.e. below heart level) at all times (to optimize perfusion)
- keeping the limb cool and exposed (reduces metabolic demand)
- close attention to daily foot washing and hygiene
- pressure relief to prevent pressure sores (especially heels)
- emollients to help prevent skin breakdown.

2.11 SUPERFICIAL THROMBOPHLEBITIS

In over 90% of cases superficial thrombophlebitis occurs in varicose veins. Statis leads to clotting within varicose veins and this can be prevented by graded elastic stockings. If superficial thrombophlebitis occurs without varicose veins it should prompt a search for occult malignancy (particularly pancreatic carcinoma), thrombocytosis or poly-thaemia. Superficial thrombophlebitis rarely leads to pulmonary embolus except when a clot propagates into the femoral vein from the long saphenous vein.

2.11.1 Treatment

Superficial thrombophlebitis below the knee should be treated with warm soaks, rest and a non-steroidal anti-inflammatory drug. Signs of inflammation abate within 5 to 10 days. For superficial thrombophlebitis in the lower thigh heparin anticoagulation is advisable. Treatment can be discontinued as soon as signs of inflammation are receding if further propagation is not evident. If the clot reaches the upper thigh, the long saphenous vein should be ligated.

FURTHER READING

Abrams WA, Beers MH and Berkow R (eds). *The Merck Manual of Geriatrics*, 2nd edn. Merck, Whitehouse Station, NJ, 1995.

British Cardiac Society Working Group/Royal College of Physicians Research Unit. *Valvular Heart Disease. Investigation and management.* Royal College of Physicians, London, 1996.

Clarke M. Cardiac pacemakers. *Prescriber J* 1993; 33:103–111.

Cohn JN. The management of chronic heart failure. *N Engl J Med* 1996; 335:490–498.

Lip GYH, Lowe GDO. Antithrombotic treatment for atrial fibrillation. *Br Med J* 1996; 312:45–49.

Martin A, Camm AJ (eds). *Geriatric Cardiology. Principles and Practice*. John Wiley & Sons, Chichester, 1994.

Mulrow CD, Cornell JA, Herrera CR et al. Hypertension in the elderly. Implications and generalizability of randomized trials. *JAMA* 1994; 272:1932–1938.

Royal College of Physicians Working Party. Cardiological interventions in elderly patients. *J Royal Coll Physicians* 1991; 25:197–205.

Sanderson S. Hypertension in the elderly: pressure to treat? *Health Trends* 1996; 28:71–75.

Scandinavian Simvastatin Survival Study Group. Randomised trial of cholesterol lowering in 4444 patients with coronary heart disease: the Scandinavian Simvastatin Survival Study (4S). *Lancet* 1994; 344:1383–1389.

Shephard J, Cobbe SM, Ford I et al. The West of Scotland Coronary Prevention Study Group. Prevention of coronary heart disease with pravastatin in men with hypercholesterolaemia. *N Engl J Med* 1995; 333:1301–1307.

Smith E, Powell H, Hastie IR. Coronary artery disease, valvular heart disease, bradycardia and heart failure. *Postgrad Med J* 1995; 71:346–353.

Staessen JA, Fagard R, Thijs L et al. (Syst-Eur Trial investigators). Randomised double-blind comparison of placebo and active treatment for older patients with isolated systolic hypertension. *Lancet* 1997; 350:757–764.

Woodhouse K, Pascual J. *Hypertension in Elderly People*. Martin Dunitz, London, 1996.

Chapter 3

Neurological Disorders

3.1 CEREBROVASCULAR DISEASE

3.1.1 Transient Ischaemic Attack

Transient ischaemic attacks (TIAs) refer to the clinical syndrome of sudden onset of neurological symptoms or signs, of cerebrovascular aetiology, which are completely resolved within 24 hours of onset. The typical features of carotid and vertebrobasilar TIA are shown in Table 3.1. Other causes of dizziness in old age are commonly misdiagnosed as TIA (Table 3.2). TIAs must be investigated urgently, since they are always warnings of possible impending stroke, the risk being highest within the first year (12%), particularly within 1 week following TIA. Transient ischaemic attack is not a diagnosis in itself, rather it is a symptom of a variety of cardiovascular disorders which can result in occlusion of cerebral vessels by thromboembolism. It is not sufficient simply to prescribe aspirin.

All patients with TIA symptoms within the previous 10 days should be investigated urgently. Clinical assessment to detect the likely underlying

Table 3.1 Typical features of transient ischaemic attack (TIA)

Carotid TIA	Vertebrobasilar TIA
Unilateral facial or limb weakness	Brainstem symptoms and signs (vertigo, diplopia, circumoral or unilateral weakness, paraesthesiae)
Unilateral facial or limb sensory alteration	Cerebellar symptoms and signs (dysarthria, ataxia, incoordination)
Dysphasia, dysarthria	
Amaurosis fugax	Homonymous hemianopia
Ipsilateral headache (in 20%)	Transient amnesia
	Occipital headache (in 20%)

Table 3.2 Other causes of dizziness frequently misdiagnosed as TIA in old age

Presyncopal lightheadedness:
 orthostatic hypotension
 vasovagal presyncope
 cardiac arrhythmias
 aortic valve disease
Labyrinthine vertigo:
 benign positional vertigo
 acute labyrinthitis
 Ménière's disease
Spondarthritis with cervical proprioceptive failure
Focal non-convulsive epilepsy
Drop attacks due to osteoarthritis of the knees
Transient global amnesia
Hypoglycaemia in diabetics
Panic attacks with hyperventilation

immediate cause of the TIA, e.g. carotid bruit, atrial fibrillation, signs of aortic or mitral valvular disease, supplemented by the relevant investigations (electrocardiogram (ECG), chest radiograph, carotid duplex ultrasound, cranial computed tomography (CT) or magnetic resonance imaging (MRI) and echocardiography as appropriate) should be carried out as soon as possible. Patients with TIA should have the same diagnostic evaluation as patients with completed stroke, looking for the major stroke risk factors (Table 3.3). Those with carotid symptoms who may be surgical candidates and have common or internal carotid stenosis of >70% on carotid ultrasound should be referred to a vascular surgeon with a view to carotid endarterectomy (CEA). Carotid angiography may be necessary in some cases to confirm high-grade carotid stenosis, but angiography is becoming less necessary as the quality and resolution of non-invasive ultrasonic imaging has greatly advanced in recent years. CEA carries a 4–5% risk of stroke compared to a 10–12% risk without surgery within 5 years. For patients with <30% carotid stenosis, CEA is not recommended and one should look for other causes of TIA. In cases of intermediate carotid stenosis (30–69%), the evidence for significant benefit from CEA versus medical therapy is unclear. However, if there is evidence of ulcerated carotid plaque and recurrent TIAs or completed small stroke(s), CEA may be justified. At present, there is no compelling evidence to support CEA in elderly people with asymptomatic high-grade carotid stenosis (>70%).

Table 3.3 Major risk factors for stroke

Previous stroke/TIA	Heavy alcohol intake	Moderate–severe COPD
Older age	Valvular heart disease	Peripheral vascular disease
Hypertension	Recent myocardial infarction	Haematocrit >50%
Atrial fibrillation	Heart failure	Carotid stenosis
Diabetes	Smoking	Marked obesity

COPD, chronic obstructive pulmonary disease.

Elderly people who are not surgical candidates should be managed with **antiplatelet therapy**. **Aspirin** (75–300 mg once daily) is effective in most patients and is well tolerated by the majority. A dose of 150 mg daily is adequate, but if dyspepsia occurs, a lower dose may be tried (usually 75 mg daily). If patients cannot take aspirin because of gastro-intestinal intolerance or allergic side-effects, **ticlopidine** (250 mg twice daily) may be used as an alternative in some countries where it is licensed. Ticlopidine exerts its antiplatelet effect by inhibition of adenosine diphosphate (ADP)-induced platelet aggregation. However, its widespread use has been limited by side-effects, principally rash, diarrhoea, nausea and vomiting. It is also associated with a 1–2% incidence of reversible neutropenia. Therefore close monitoring of full blood counts every 2 weeks for the first 3 months is essential for ticlopidine therapy. The drug should be stopped if the absolute neutro-phil count falls below 1000 cells/µl. **Clopidogrel** is chemically similar to ticlopidine, is equally effective as an antiplatelet agent and appears to be safer. The value of other antiplatelet agents (e.g. dipyridamole, sulphinpyrazone) in primary stroke prevention is unclear and they are not currently recommended, although there is some evidence that modified-release dipyridamole (200 mg twice daily) may be more beneficial for *secondary* stroke prevention than low-dose aspirin alone. Modified-release dipyridamole may also have a role in patients following TIA who cannot tolerate aspirin.

Warfarin is no better than aspirin for patients with TIA, and is not recommended first-line therapy for patients who are in sinus rhythm. However, in patients who continue to have TIAs due to atheromatous plaque fissure despite adequate antiplatelet therapy and where endarter-ectomy is not indicated, heparin followed by warfarin for 1–3 months may be given, although evidence of significant benefit in such cases is lacking. Following 1–3 months' warfarin therapy, antiplatelet therapy may be restarted. Equally important in TIA management is risk factor modification, as for secondary stroke prevention (see section 3.1.6).

3.1.2   Assessment of Risk Factors for Stroke

Stroke is the single greatest cause of major physical disability in Western countries. Although the mortality from stroke has fallen in the last 30 years, it is unclear whether the **incidence** of stroke is declining. This is because of the current demographic trend towards increasing proportions of elderly people in the population and the fact that stroke is an age-related disorder. Also, the proportion of people with stroke disease who are elderly is increasing. In the USA, the proportion of persons with stroke disease who were over 65 increased significantly from 67% in the late 1940s to 77% in the early 1980s. Stroke is defined by rapidly developing clinical symptoms and/or signs of focal or global loss of cerebral function, with symptoms lasting more than 24 hours or leading to death in less than 24 hours, with no apparent cause other than a vascular one. The clinical assessment of stroke patients aims to define and quantify the motor, sensory, cognitive and psychological impairments and disabilities as well as to identify and anticipate any complications. Risk factors must be identified with a view to secondary prevention (see Table 3.2).

3.1.3   Investigation of Stroke Patients

The following tests are **required in all stroke patients**: erythrocyte sedimentation rate, full blood count, serum urea and electrolytes, blood glucose, prothrombin time and ECG. **Cranial CT or MRI** should be done in all cases to establish the diagnosis, and should be done urgently where there is:

- uncertainty about the diagnosis, particularly in comatose cases
- suspicion of condition that requires neurosurgical intervention, i.e. subarachnoid haemorrhage, cerebellar or primary intracerebral haematoma, secondary hydrocephalus or subdural haematoma

- a need to exclude intracranial bleeding in order to start urgent anticoagulant therapy (e.g. proven pulmonary embolus).

Unenhanced CT imaging does not usually show small or moderately sized ischaemic cerebral infarcts clearly until about 48 hours have elapsed from the onset of the stroke ictus, but cerebral haemorrhages will be detectable immediately. If haemorrhage is discovered on brain imaging, antiplatelet and anticoagulant therapy should be withheld. As with TIA, **carotid duplex ultrasound** imaging should be performed in selected cases where

- there is a clear history of a carotid territory ischaemic stroke
- there is good functional recovery
- patients are suitable for CEA (i.e. surgery not contraindicated).

The absence of a carotid bruit does not exclude high-grade carotid stenosis. Similarly, the presence of a carotid bruit does not indicate the degree of stenosis. Patients with confirmed high-grade stenoses ($>70\%$) on ultrasound should be referred 4–6 weeks after the stroke to an experienced vascular surgeon for CEA assessment. The role of carotid angioplasty for primary and secondary stroke prevention is unclear and there is no evidence at present to support its use outside randomized controlled trials.

A variety of additional investigations in selected stroke patients may be appropriate. **Echocardiography** is indicated in cases with a suspected intracardiac source of embolism, e.g.

- atrial fibrillation (AF)
- myocardial infarction in the previous 3 months
- prosthetic valve
- suspected or known mitral or aortic valvular disease
- suspected endocarditis.

MRI may be useful in defining brainstem and posterior fossa lesions where there is clinical or radiological uncertainty. MRI also allows distinction between haemorrhagic and ischaemic lesions several weeks after the stroke, which is an advantage over CT imaging. **Lumbar**

puncture is necessary in cases where there is clinical suspicion of subarachnoid haemorrhage (neck stiffness, history of sudden onset of headache) and unenhanced CT imaging is inconclusive. **Thyroid function tests** are indicated only in those with confirmed AF or suspected thyroid disease.

3.1.4   Immediate Management of Stroke Patients

There are no drug therapies aimed at reducing the extent of cerebral infarction that are proven safe and effective for the majority of acute stroke patients. Such therapies include unfractionated heparin, corticosteroids for cerebral oedema, haemodilution techniques for improving cerebral perfusion, nimodipine and other calcium antagonists to prevent calcium influx into neurones, N-methyl-D-aspartate (NMDA) receptor antagonists etc. Routine thrombolysis is associated with **increased** morbidity and mortality and cannot be recommended, except in occasional cases where symptoms have begun less than 3 hours previously and haemorrhagic stroke has been excluded on imaging. Tissue plasminogen activator (tPA) is recommended for this indication in the USA. Therefore, emphasis is on prevention of complications (Table 3.4).

3.1.5   Management of Immediate Stroke Complications

Raised blood pressure (BP) following stroke is common and represents a reflex response by the brain to restore perfusion to the ischaemic territory, since the brain has a low resistance circulation that is dependent on systemic perfusion pressure. After most strokes, BP settles gradually to pre-stroke levels without treatment over the course of the first 7–10 days. Because of the risk of causing extension of the initial stroke, raised BP (i.e. systolic BP up to 220 mmHg ± diastolic BP up to 120 mmHg) immediately after stroke in the majority of cases should **not** be lowered. There are occasional circumstances associated with stroke where hypertension must be treated immediately, i.e.

- left ventricular failure
- hypertensive encephalopathy (drowsiness, seizures)

Table 3.4 Management and prevention of non-neurological complications of acute stroke

Dehydration: 2–3 litres of fluid daily, by intravenous infusion if patient is dysphagic.
Aspiration pneumonia: 'nil by mouth' order if confirmed/suspected dysphagia or confirmed dysphagia following assessment by speech and language therapist.
Deep vein thrombosis/pulmonary embolism: below-knee elastic stockings (avoid low-dose heparin).
Pressure sores: regular turning, skin hygiene, pressure relieving mattresses, attention to nutrition and continence.
Constipation/faecal impaction/faecal incontinence: sufficient fibre in diet, laxatives or suppositories as needed.
Urinary tract infection: aim for regular bladder drainage; avoid indwelling bladder catheters if possible.
Urinary incontinence: regular toileting, prevention of faecal impaction, penile sheath in males, absorbent pads, oxybutinin in selected cases. Use bladder catheters as a last resort.
Falls and injuries: assess safety of transfers, walking gait and awareness of hazards. Avoid restraints and use bed-rails only as a last resort.
Painful shoulder: careful positioning and prophylactic arm support for all patients with flaccid hemiplegias.
Limb contractures: weekly checks of passive range of movement, therapy of associated pain or anxiety.
Hiccoughs: may be persistent and distressing in patients with brainstem strokes. Empiric therapy with phenothiazines (e.g. chlorpromazine 25 mg twice daily) or anticonvulsants may be tried. Observe for hypotension with phenothiazines.

- progressive acute renal failure
- acute aortic dissection.

In these situations, BP should be reduced **gradually** to target levels of 140 mmHg for systolic BP and 95 mmHg for diastolic BP. A beta-blocker (e.g. metoprolol) is a suitable first choice drug, unless contra-indicated. Some authorities recommend using intravenous labetalol or nitroprusside with careful monitoring of BP, as for accelerated hypertension. However, it is best not to lower BP aggressively in the first few days after stroke **unless** there is underlying accelerated hypertension. Patients with known hypertension who are already on treatment should continue on their medication, provided they can swallow their tablets.

Epileptic seizures should be terminated in the usual way with rectal or intravenous diazepam. **Prolonged seizures must be avoided** to prevent further increase of infarct volume, as occurs in animal models of acute stroke. It is advisable to start prophylactic anticonvulsant therapy after a single seizure in acute stroke (see section 3.2), since the recurrence rate is at least 50% in the first year after stroke.

Pyrexia is also likely to lead to increased infarct volume since raised core body temperature increases metabolic demand in the ischaemic penumbral zone. Aspiration pneumonia and urinary tract infection are particularly likely to cause pyrexia in the first few days following acute stroke. Pyrexia may also result from severe ischaemic stroke or subarachnoid haemorrhage affecting hypothalamic thermoregulation. Therefore, it is recommended that pyrexia should be treated with paracetamol (by suppository if necessary), and appropriate antibiotic therapy where indicated. Aspiration pneumonia should be treated in the usual way, with antibiotics, physiotherapy and supplemental oxygen. Further episodes should be prevented by adopting appropriate feeding strategies, based on a swallowing assessment and the recommendations of the speech and language therapist.

Hyperglycaemia is commonly seen in acute stroke, either as a result of poorly controlled diabetes mellitus or as a stress response in more severe strokes. It is associated with poorer outcome and reduced survival. Although there are no randomized, controlled studies of careful normalization of blood glucose in acute stroke, blood glucose concentration should probably be corrected to between 4 and 8 mmol/l, by insulin and dextrose infusion if necessary.

3.1.6 Secondary Prevention of Stroke

Antiplatelet therapy is indicated for all patients with acute ischaemic stroke who are in sinus rhythm. **Aspirin** (160–300 mg once daily) started within 48 hours of stroke onset has been shown to result in approximately 10 fewer deaths in the first 2–4 weeks per 1000 patients treated, and about 13 fewer patients dead or dependent per 1000 treated after 6 months. Aspirin may be given by suppository in dysphagic patients, if necessary. Aspirin may be started immediately, but exclusion of haemorrhagic stroke by CT scanning is desirable, in order to minimize the risk of an excess of deaths from haemorrhagic strokes. **Anticoagulation** with warfarin prevents about 90 serious vascular events (mostly strokes) per 1000 patients with AF and a previous TIA or stroke in one year, i.e. about 11 TIA or stroke survivors need to be treated with anticoagulants for one year to prevent one vascular event (stroke, myocardial infarct, systemic embolism or cardiovascular death). Warfarin is more effective than aspirin (which is better than placebo) and should be prescribed in all patients in AF, **unless there is a contraindication**, such as:

- uncontrolled hypertension
- dementia
- frequent falls (risk of cerebral and other major bleeding)
- poor drug compliance or difficulty with monitoring international normalized ratio (INR)
- bleeding disorders of any kind, or
- infective endocarditis.

Age per se is not a contraindication to warfarin after first stroke. Treatment may be started 2 weeks after an ischaemic stroke and should be life-long, with the INR adjusted to 2.0–3.0. Warfarin should be given for 3–6 months in patients in sinus rhythm, whose strokes were associated with recent myocardial infarction. Further systemic thromboembolism in such patients should be followed by life-long anticoagulation. Similarly, patients with rapidly advancing neurological deficit (so-called '**stroke in evolution**') should be considered for full anticoagulation with heparin, followed by warfarin for 3–6 months.

Carotid endarterectomy (CEA) is recommended in surgically fit patients following carotid territory TIA or minor stroke with confirmed high-grade carotid stenosis (70–99%) on carotid angiography. CEA reduces the risk of death or stroke in the 3-year period after surgery from approximately 22% (with medical therapy alone) to approximately 12%. About 5% of patients undergoing CEA have a stroke or die within 1 month of surgery, but this risk does not outweigh the benefit of CEA in high-risk patients.

Antihypertensive therapy is recommended for patients with sustained systolic BP >160 mmHg and/or diastolic BP >100 mmHg, where successful reduction of salt, alcohol and body weight have not been effective in correcting raised BP. Thiazides and beta-blockers are suitable first-line drugs, as with primary stroke prevention.

Cessation of smoking should be advised in all patients following TIA or stroke. Additional measures such as nicotine patches and support groups may be helpful in achieving this aim.

Diabetic control should be stringent but not over-rigorous to avoid the dangers of hypoglycaemia in stroke patients.

Hyperlipidaemia has a more important aetiological role in coronary heart disease than in cerebrovascular disease, and any benefit from lipid-lowering therapy in elderly patients following TIA or stroke is, as yet, unclear. Nevertheless, the use of statins to reduce cholesterol in secondary prevention studies (mostly coronary heart disease), is associated with a reduction in the risk of stroke of about 30%. At the moment, the evidence is not sufficiently strong to recommend cholesterol-reducing therapy in all elderly patients following stroke or TIA.

3.1.7 Chronic Stroke Complications

Depression is noted in approximately 45% of patients after stroke, about half of whom meet diagnostic criteria for major depression. Ten to 15% of stroke survivors will have persistent, significant depression when followed up 2 years after their stroke. Post-stroke depression may be particularly difficult to diagnose if the patient has communication problems. It should be distinguished from post-stroke emotionalism and apathy due to right hemispheric infarction. Depression may be a major obstacle to rehabilitation progress and careful monitoring of mood is essential. Where doubt exists, a trial of antidepressant therapy is usually indicated. There is no good evidence that any one class of antidepressant is any better than another in this situation. However, some caution is necessary with tricyclic antidepressants in patients with constipation and bladder dysfunction as a result of their stroke, and selective serotonin reuptake inhibitors may therefore be preferable to tricyclic drugs as first-line therapy. In severe post-stroke depression that does not respond to medication, electroconvulsive therapy has been used effectively and safely.

Spasticity sets in after several weeks to months following hemiplegic stroke. It is often distressing due to associated pain, deformity and disability. It may lead to secondary pressure sores, e.g. medial aspect of the knee with thigh adductor spasticity, and eventually irreversible limb-deforming contractures. Physiotherapy aims to modulate tone in the affected limb and the more a hemiplegic patient is able to use his/her affected side, the lower the risk of spasticity. Concurrent anxiety and pain in the affected limb increase muscle tone and the risk of spasticity, so treatment of these underlying problems is helpful. Traditional '**anti-spasticity' drugs** (baclofen, dantrolene and diazepam) are occasionally helpful, but elderly patients are less tolerant to their side-effects (sedation, hypotonia and muscle weakness) than younger patients. Local injection of **botulinum toxin** has been reported to be beneficial in troublesome spasticity, is easy to administer but is expensive.

Malnutrition after stroke may occur for a variety of reasons, principally persistent dysphagia, sepsis, depression and poor nursing care. Nutritional supplements in the form of high calorie, high protein drinks are helpful in patients who can swallow. Patients at risk of aspiration may require fine-bore **nasogastric tube** feeding, which should not be delayed beyond 48–72 hours after the ictus, provided tube feeding is appropriate. Competence in swallowing should be assessed on a daily basis by a trained person (e.g. speech and language therapist or specialist nurse) who can advise on whether swallowing is 'safe' or not, and if it is, what the most appropriate form of oral intake should be. **Percutaneous endoscopic gastrostomy** (PEG) tube feeding is usually held in reserve for the small minority (1–2%) of stroke patients whose dysphagia is severe and persistent beyond 14 days. Careful patient selection is the key to optimal use of PEG tube feeding, and there is no reason to stop swallowing rehabilitation when a PEG tube is inserted. PEG tube feeding should be avoided in patients with impaired conscious level or with a low probability of survival beyond the first month after stroke.

Urinary incontinence affects one-third to a half of all post-stroke patients. Causes include:

- impaired conscious level or confusion
- detrusor instability
- immobility
- undressing disability or dyspraxia
- inability to manage urinal bottles or a commode
- urinary tract infection

- bladder outflow obstruction due to prostatism or faecal impaction
- polyuria due to diuretic therapy or hyperglycaemia.

Identification and correction of underlying cause(s) may cure the problem (see also section 10.2).

Faecal incontinence is usually due to continuing impaired conscious or cognitive level, or constipation with faecal impaction/overflow diarrhoea. Regular laxative suppositories or enemas are helpful in patients with impaired conscious level and are also useful in the short term to treat faecal impaction. Increased dietary fibre and judicious use of oral laxatives usually abolish faecal incontinence where constipation is the underlying problem.

Pressure sores are usually preventable with good nursing care, frequent change of posture and appropriate pressure-relieving devices (see also section 13.1).

Painful shoulder affects about one-third of patients after stroke, mostly on the hemiparetic side with symptoms usually appearing in the first week. Most cases are caused by stretching of the joint capsule from the weight of the unsupported upper limb or by excessive traction force during assisted posture transfers. Careful positioning and support of the arm as well as shoulder slings that avoid flexion of the elbow and wrist are helpful, and care must be taken to avoid pulling on the affected limb. Activities that cause shoulder pain should be minimized, but this must be balanced by passive shoulder movements to avoid onset of 'frozen shoulder' (adhesive capsulitis). Non-steroidal anti-inflammatory drugs, local and systemic corticosteroids, tricyclic antidepressants and anti-spasticity drugs have been tried with modest success. Non-pharmacological methods such as ultrasound and transcutaneous electrical stimulation (TENS) are also worth trying.

Swollen, cold arms may result from gravitational oedema in a dependent limb, poor muscle tone and power, unrecognized injury and reflex sympathetic dystrophy. Reflex sympathetic dystrophy refers to a group of idiopathic disorders characterized by persistent pain, altered sensation, sudomotor and vasomotor changes and bone/soft tissue dystrophy leading to major loss of limb function. The same factors may cause swollen, cold legs but other causes such as deep vein thrombosis, cardiac failure and hypoalbuminaemia should be considered. Where gravitational oedema is the cause, treatment should include elevation, graduated compression and encouragement of active movement where possible.

3.2 EPILEPSY

The incidence of seizure disorder increases markedly after late middle age in parallel to the steep rise in the incidence of cerebrovascular disease, principally established stroke. The causes of epilepsy in old age differ in type and incidence from younger people, as listed in Table 3.5. A good witness account is the best aid to diagnosis, but where doubt exists, structural brain imaging (CT or MRI) is helpful, since structural abnormalities and evidence of cerebrovascular disease support the diagnosis of epilepsy. Electroencephalography (EEG) is of doubtful value in the diagnosis of epilepsy in elderly people, since a normal EEG does not exclude epilepsy, and non-specific EEG abnormalities are common in old age. Epilepsy must be distinguished from non-epileptic events, such as syncope, drop attacks, TIAs, hypoglycaemia, paroxysmal behaviour disturbances associated with dementia and transient global amnesia. Useful indicators of seizure include sudden onset without warning, urinary incontinence, post-ictal confusional state and significant injury. Distinction of a fit from a faint (syncope) may be difficult in

Table 3.5 Common causes of epilepsy in old age compared with younger adults

Old age	Younger adults
Cerebrovascular disease and stroke	Idiopathic
Intracranial tumour (metastatic)	Head injury
Syncope, global cerebral ischaemia	Intracerebral, subarachnoid bleeding
Metabolic disorders (hypoglycaemia, hypoxia, hyponatraemia, hypothyroidism, hypocalcaemia)	Infection (meningitis, encephalitis)
	Primary brain tumour
Severe organ failure (hepatic, renal failure)	Drug overdose (e.g. tricyclic antidepressants)
Drugs (e.g. theophylline, doxapram, anticholinergics)	Drug withdrawal (e.g. ethanol, benzodiazepines, opioids)
Drug withdrawal states (e.g. ethanol, benzodiazepines)	Metabolic disorders

elderly people, given that secondary seizures with syncope are not uncommon and the fact that the event is less likely to be witnessed in an elderly person. Seizures may also be misdiagnosed as other clinical problems that occur more commonly in old age, such as Parkinson's disease (continuous partial epilepsy), TIA (sensory epilepsy), hemiparetic stroke (Todd's paresis), confusional state (complex partial status epilepsy), and falls (seizures of any type).

Before considering the pharmacological aspects of epilepsy management in old age, the often neglected non-pharmacological aspects must be stressed. The patient and his/her family need information about the condition and the main restrictions a diagnosis of epilepsy brings with it, e.g. bathing, driving, alcohol intake. Elderly epileptics who live alone are particularly vulnerable so that assessment of the home environment by an occupational therapist and social support are important considerations. Where appropriate, the elderly patient should also be put in contact with the local branches of national support agencies, e.g. the British Epilepsy Association, for information and support.

There is broad agreement that adults require anticonvulsant therapy after two or more unprovoked major seizures (recurrence rate approximately 70%). At present, there are no published large, randomized controlled trials that have addressed the issue of whether treatment should be started after a single generalized seizure, and general consensus about this issue is lacking. However, if there is an obvious seizure-provoking pathology, such as stroke or tumour, or the risks of serious injury (particularly hip fracture) from further seizures are considered high, therapy may be warranted after a first seizure. The first-line, broad-spectrum anticonvulsants for primary generalized, secondary generalized and partial seizures are **phenytoin**, **carbamazepine** and **sodium valproate**. The aim of therapy is complete control of seizures on the lowest effective dose of a single first-line drug. The three first-line drugs have approximately equal efficacy and tolerability, and all have the potential to cause **non-specific neurological side-effects** of drowsiness, cerebellar dysfunction, dizziness, blurred or double vision and asterixis. Similarly, all three drugs can result in chronic cognitive impairment but this problem is minimized if doses are kept to the lowest effective level. Non-neurological side-effects and compliance may influence which first-line drug is selected (Table 3.6). The saturation kinetics of phenytoin

Table 3.6 Pharmacology of first-line anticonvulsants

	Phenytoin	Carbamazepine	Sodium valproate
Starting dose	200 mg	100 mg b.i.d.	200 mg b.i.d.
Daily maintenance dose	200–300 mg o.d.	600–1200 mg (b.i.d. or t.i.d. dose)	1000–2000 mg (b.i.d. or t.i.d. dose)
Plasma half-life (elderly)	Unknown	Unknown	11–17 hours
Metabolism	Hepatic	Hepatic	Hepatic
Active metabolites	None	Yes	Unknown
Idiosyncratic toxicity	Rash, hepatitis, skin, gum hypertrophy folate deficiency, lymphadenopathy, osteomalacia	Transient leucopenia, hyponatraemia, rash	Dyspepsia, vomiting, transient alopecia, hepatitis, false positive ketonuria, acute pancreatitis
Therapeutic plasma levels	10–20 μg/ml	4–12 μg/ml	50–100 μg/ml

o.d., daily; b.i.d., twice daily; t.i.d., three times daily.

mean that dose increments in the higher end of the therapeutic range may result in toxic levels, unless they are limited to 25–50 mg at a time. First-line anticonvulsants should be started at the lower end of the therapeutic range and dosages increased gradually, unless seizures are frequent and possibly life-threatening. Routine monitoring of plasma drug levels is not recommended and the correct dose of anticonvulsant is the lowest effective dose, regardless of whether the plasma level is in the 'therapeutic range' or not. Plasma anticonvulsant levels may be helpful where:

- compliance is doubtful
- seizure control is poor, despite good compliance (to ensure that adequate plasma levels are being reached, before deciding on a dose increase or changing to another drug)
- dose increments of phenytoin at the upper end of the dose range are needed, and
- drug toxicity is suspected.

Phenytoin and carbamazepine are powerful liver enzyme inducing agents, so that the metabolism of concurrently prescribed drugs may be accelerated, e.g. warfarin, with serious consequences. Therefore, when starting anticonvulsant therapy or any other drug when anti-convulsants are being prescribed, a careful check should be made for possible adverse drug interactions.

Occasionally, seizure control in older patients may be poor, so-called **'brittle epilepsy'**. This relates to the fact that most epilepsy in old age is secondary to focal cerebral infarction of variable size and location, readily leading to partial epilepsy with or without secondary generalization. Provided compliance and plasma drug levels have been optimized, the dose of the first-line, broad-spectrum anticonvulsant should be gradually increased to the maximum tolerated level. If seizure control is still inadequate, a second first-line drug may be introduced, whilst the first agent is gradually withdrawn. The dose of the second drug should be steadily increased to the usual maintenance level or to the maximum tolerated level, if the patient still experiences seizures. Although a third first-line drug may be tried as monotherapy, if the other two first-line agents have failed, many clinicians add **gabapentin**, **topiramate**, **vigabatrin** or **lamotrigine** to a first-line drug in cases of poorly controlled seizures.

Other anticonvulsant drugs for long-term use, such as barbiturates and benzodiazepines, do not have a significant role in the modern management of epilepsy in old age, and should be avoided. Sometimes, however, elderly patients may be encountered who have been taking barbiturate anticonvulsants for many years, without seizures in the previous 3 years and apparently without adverse drug side-effects. Provided seizure control is satisfactory and the patient does not manifest signs of drug toxicity, it is wise not to alter therapy.

3.3 PARKINSONISM

Approximately 1% of all people over the age of 60 in Western countries have Parkinsonism. Of these, 80–90% suffer from idiopathic Parkinson's disease, the classical features of which are listed in Table 3.7. However, Parkinson's disease is misdiagnosed in approximately 20% of cases, even when clinical diagnostic criteria are carefully applied, as confirmed by autopsy studies. The conditions most commonly misdiagnosed as Parkinson's disease are:

Table 3.7 Classical clinical features of idiopathic Parkinson's disease

* Parkinsonian syndrome (i.e. bradykinesia plus one or more of the following: muscular rigidity, resting tremor, postural instability) *plus* at least 3 of the following features:
* Unilateral onset
* Resting tremor
* Progressive disorder
* Persistent asymmetry affecting the side of onset more
* Excellent response to levodopa
* Levodopa-induced dyskinesias
* Levodopa response for 5 years or more
* Clinical course for 10 years or more

- essential tremor
- 'senile gait'
- cerebrovascular Parkinsonism
- drug-induced Parkinsonism and
- multi-system atrophy (including striatonigral degeneration, Shy–Drager syndrome, progressive supranuclear palsy).

The clinical features of these Parkinsonian syndromes are detailed in Table 3.8. They are sometimes referred to as 'Parkinson's-plus' syndromes, i.e. Parkinsonism in addition to other neurological features, not typical of idiopathic Parkinson's disease. It is important to ascertain the 'Parkinson's-plus' syndromes, since they do not respond well to dopaminergic therapy and therefore have a worse prognosis. One of the most useful things to know at the outset is whether there is a significant improvement to a test dose of levodopa (e.g. co-careldopa 100/25 mg). The initial response to levodopa is a strong predictor of continued benefit from therapy at 1 month. Patients with a poor response to the initial test dose usually do not have idiopathic Parkinson's disease (i.e. long-term levodopa responsiveness).

There are important differences between young (<50 years) and older (>70 years) patients with idiopathic Parkinson's disease (IPD). Motor fluctuations and dyskinesia, which occur early and tend to be severe in young patients, are generally late and mild in older patients. Actuarial life expectancy is measured in decades in young patients, but is much shorter in older patients, so IPD manifesting *de novo* in old age seldom

Table 3.8   Pseudo-Parkinson's syndromes: clinical features

(i) Essential tremor
Symmetrical, worse with movement, often familial (autosomal dominant), titubation frequently, macrographia, not relieved by anti-Parkinsonian therapy

(ii) Senile gait
Shuffling gait, transient freezing of legs, absence of Parkinsonian features above the waist

(iii) Cerebrovascular Parkinsonism
Upper motor neurone or sensory long tract signs or extensor plantar responses, prominent cerebrovascular risk factors (particularly hypertension)

(iv) Drug-induced Parkinsonism
Therapy with the following: neuroleptics, prochlorperazine, metoclopramide, methyldopa, cinnarizine, lithium, fluoxetine, calcium antagonists
Coincidence with starting drug therapy, symmetrical Parkinsonian features, resting tremor less prominent

(v) Multisystem atrophy
Parkinsonism that is symmetrical, absence of or low-grade resting tremor
Cerebellar or pyramidal tract signs or both
Prominent early autonomic failure (e.g. marked postural hypotension, bladder dysfunction) and/or dementia
Impaired voluntary (particularly vertical) eye movements; reflex eye movements (e.g. doll's eye) intact
Pseudobulbar palsy
Posture classically not flexed as in idiopathic Parkinson's disease
Absent, poor or transient response to levodopa
Relatively rapid clinical deterioration (within 2–3 years of symptom onset)

(vi) Lewy Body disease
Dementia
Parkinsonism
Vivid hallucinations (usually visual, not drug-related)
Fluctuating clinical course

runs its full course. Cognitive impairment is rare in young patients, but affects 20–30% of elderly patients with IPD. Anticholinergics and multiple drug regimens are generally well tolerated by young patients, but are poorly tolerated by elderly patients.

In general, elderly patients with IPD should **start levodopa therapy as soon as symptom control is needed**, since there is less concern about the long-term side-effects of levodopa than in young patients. **Selegiline,**

the selective monoamine oxidase-B enzyme inhibitor, is of doubtful benefit and is not proven to be neuroprotective (as was suggested by early research studies). **Anticholinergics (e.g. benzhexol, orphenadrine, benztropine) should be avoided** in older patients because of the high risk of side-effects, particularly confusion, constipation and bladder problems. **Amantadine and dopamine agonists (e.g. bromocriptine, pergolide, lisuride) should only be used with caution in elderly IPD patients (if at all)**, because of increased risk of side-effects (nausea, vomiting, confusion, hypotension). Chronic cognitive impairment is three to four times more prevalent in elderly patients with IPD and elderly cognitively impaired patients should only have levodopa for their motor disability. The role of the new catechol-*O*-methyltransferase inhibitors (e.g. entacapone, tolcapone), which enhance dopamine effects by inhibiting its metabolism, in the management of elderly IPD cases is unclear, although trials in younger IPD patients indicate efficacy.

The **common adverse effects of levodopa** include:

- orthostatic hypotension
- nausea and vomiting
- delirium and hallucinations
- involuntary movements (dystonic reactions).

Less commonly, there may be:

- cardiac arrhythmias
- sweating
- dark urine
- constipation.

To minimize side-effects, levodopa is given in the lowest effective dose. In general, it is reasonable to start with 50–100 mg levodopa (e.g. as co-beneldopa) every 4 hours up to bedtime. If patients cannot change their posture in bed and have insomnia as a result, a sustained-release levodopa preparation (100–200 mg) at bedtime is appropriate. If patients find themselves akinetic in the morning despite a bedtime dose of levodopa, dispersible levodopa (e.g. co-beneldopa) is usually helpful to produce a rapid switch-on of voluntary movement. Usually, elderly patients do well with levodopa therapy in the first 1–2 years. Later, however, many patients develop motor fluctuations or drug-induced dyskinesia (involuntary movements). End-of-dose deterioration and so-called 'on–off' fluctuation of akinesia are commonly seen, the 'on–off' effect following end-of-dose deterioration as the disease progresses. In the later stages of IPD, patients may also experience involuntary dyskinetic movements, and psychiatric side-effects associated with levodopa dose escalation (e.g. nightmares, illusions, pseudohallucinations, mood swings and behavioural disturbances). Table 3.9 details the management of levodopa-related complications.

Amantadine may be tried in occasional patients who cannot tolerate levodopa or who present with very mild symptoms. It works by enhancing dopamine release from storage vesicles in dopaminergic nerve endings. The usual dose is 100 mg twice daily. It may be associated with livedo reticularis, peripheral oedema and psychosis. **Dopamine receptor agonists (bromocriptine, pergolide, lisuride, ropinirole)** work principally by stimulating D2 receptors in the corpus striatum. They may be useful occasionally for nocturnal akinesia, where levodopa alone is ineffective or poorly tolerated, or where attempting to manage 'off' phenomena with levodopa adjustment has been unsuccessful. There is little advantage with one dopamine agonist drug over another. **Bromocriptine** is usually started at a dose of 2.5 mg at bedtime and gradually increased to a dose of 10–40 mg daily as a three or four times daily regimen. Each of the dopamine agonists is associated with nausea through stimulation of dopamine receptors in the medullary chemoreceptor trigger zone. Bromocriptine is also associated with orthostatic hypotension, abdominal discomfort, constipation, blurred vision, Raynaud's phenomenon, ankle oedema and rarely retroperitoneal fibrosis. Nausea and postural hypotension may be treated with the peripherally acting dopamine receptor antagonist, **domperidone** (10–20 mg three times daily).

Apomorphine, which can only be given parenterally, has recently been rediscovered as a useful drug in end-stage IPD. It stimulates D1 and D2 receptors and may be very useful in patients who experience severe or unpredictable motor fluctuations. Apomorphine is highly reliable, usually giving relief of akinesia within 15 minutes of subcutaneous (0.5–4 mg) injection, and is therefore a very useful 'rescue' device. It may be conveniently given intermittently in anticipation or at the onset of 'off' periods using an injection device which is easily loaded with

Table 3.9 Management of levodopa-related complications in Parkinson's disease

(a) End-of-dose deterioration
Try smaller doses of levodopa more frequently *or*
Try a controlled-release (CR) levodopa preparation with additional standard levodopa to 'kick start' akinesia (most patients require 3–4-hourly CR levodopa).
Try cautious low-dose bromocriptine if levodopa dose manipulation has failed and symptoms are severe.

(b) Nocturnal akinesia
Try CR levodopa at bedtime.
Try a dopamine agonist at bedtime, if levodopa does not work, and bromocriptine is tolerated.

(c) Postprandial akinesia
Try restricting protein intake to the evening meal (the large neutral amino acids use the same gut transport system as levodopa, and may competitively block levodopa absorption).

(d) Severe, unpredictable fluctuations, unresponsive to levodopa manipulation or orally active dopamine agonists
Consider subcutaneous apomorphine infusion pump (following premedication with domperidone for 72 hours).

(e) Peak dose dyskinesias
Try smaller doses of levodopa more frequently.
If unsuccessful or the patient experiences severe 'on–off' periods, try partial replacement of levodopa therapy with a dopamine agonist (try bromocriptine first, with its short duration of action).

(f) 'Off period' dystonic spasms
Try dispersible levodopa (e.g. co-beneldopa) for more rapid effect than levodopa tablets.
If unsuccessful, try CR levodopa (to avoid levodopa concentration troughs), with a 'kick start' dose of dispersible levodopa in the morning.
If unsuccessful, try partial replacement of levodopa with dopamine agonist.
If unsuccessful, consider apomorphine subcutaneous injection or infusion.
If unsuccessful, try baclofen.

(g) Acute levodopa-related confusional state or behaviour disorder
Try smaller doses more frequently. Once the problem is resolved or attenuated, try CR levodopa to avoid levodopa concentration peaks.

cartridges containing fixed doses of drug. However, its effects are short-lived (40–70 minutes). In carefully selected elderly patients, this problem may be overcome by giving the drug as a continuous subcutaneous infusion, driven by a portable battery-operated infusion pump, with concurrent oral domperidone to counteract the nausea/vomiting.

However, this form of therapy needs to be supervised by a physician or a nurse with appropriate expertise. Subcutaneous apomorphine therapy may be associated with bleeding, abscesses, subcutaneous nodules and pigmentation at injection/infusion sites. These problems are minimized by rotating the injection site on a daily basis. Rarely, autoimmune haemolytic anaemia results from apomorphine therapy. Full blood counts every 4–6 months are therefore recommended.

There are **some practices in the treatment of elderly patients with IPD that are best avoided** (Table 3.10). Stereotactic surgery is seldom appropriate in elderly patients with end-stage IPD, where levodopa therapy no longer works, not least because of lack of convincing evidence of efficacy and safety. The same applies to neural tissue transplantation.

Psychiatric problems occur commonly in patients with IPD. Major depression affects 30–40% of patients at some stage in their illness. **Tricyclic antidepressants** should be the first choice therapy, unless there are contraindications or tricyclic therapy is poorly tolerated (e.g. causing severe, treatment-resistant constipation), in which case selective serotonin reuptake inhibitor therapy may be tried. Delirium is not uncommon in elderly IPD patients, and anti-Parkinsonian drugs are often the culprits. If the patient is taking multiple anti-Parkinsonian drugs, the last drug added to the regimen should be stopped first. If IPD patients manifest psychosis that does not respond to rationalizing drug therapy, and if neuroleptic therapy becomes necessary, **risperidone** or

Table 3.10 Practices to be avoided in the treatment of elderly patients with idiopathic Parkinson's disease

---

(1) Levodopa therapy when there is no disability in the early stages of IPD.
(2) Starting regular levodopa therapy without confirming levodopa responsiveness.
(3) Standard levodopa as once or twice daily therapy, with the assumption that elderly patients need less (it is usually required every 3–4 hours).
(4) Drug 'holidays' (associated with increased morbidity and mortality).
(5) Unsuitable neuroleptics (such as thioridazine, chlorpromazine, haloperidol) for agitated or confused patients (risk of severe akinetic state which may be fatal as a result of falls, pressure sores, pneumonia).
(6) Adding on each class of anti-Parkinsonian drug, when levodopa therapy has failed (toxicity likely).

olanzapine may be cautiously introduced (see section 5.1). Conventional neuroleptics are to be avoided in demented Parkinsonian patients.

Finally, adjunctive **physiotherapy and speech/swallowing therapy should be considered at each stage of the disease**, although for sustained benefit, therapy may need to be continuous. Also, an **occupational therapist** should assess the need for home equipment to optimize independent living, a need that is underestimated in IPD. Counselling and support of patients and their carers (e.g. by the Parkinson's Disease Society in the UK), is paramount, particularly when the diagnosis is first made.

3.4   DIZZINESS AND 'FUNNY TURNS'

Dizziness means different things to different people, particularly elderly people. It is usually taken to mean a sensation of light-headedness or unsteadiness. It is the single greatest reason for elderly patients (particularly those over 75 years) consulting their general practitioner. Elderly patients with dizziness or 'funny turns' are commonly misdiagnosed as having TIAs (see Table 3.2). The first task is to define exactly what the patient means by dizziness. Usually, it means syncope due to global cerebral hypoperfusion or vertigo with an illusion of tilting or rotatory movement or a fear of falling in those with a history of falls or balance problems. The **most important causes of syncopal dizziness** are:

- age-related orthostatic hypotension
- hypotensive drugs
- vasovagal syncope
- arrhythmias
- low output cardiac failure
- aortic valvular disease (see also Chapter 2).

Orthostatic hypotension (OH) is said to exist when there is a fall of >20 mmHg in systolic blood pressure from the supine to the standing posture. Once causative drugs have been excluded, the commonest cause of this problem is thought to be an age-related impairment of baroreflex function. Interestingly, many elderly people with OH have isolated systolic hypertension, and the height of the supine systolic BP is the most accurate predictor of the degree of OH. The drugs that commonly

Table 3.11   Drugs commonly associated with orthostatic hypotension and dizziness

Diuretics (loop and thiazide)
Vasodilators (nitrates, calcium channel blockers, alpha-1 antagonists, ACE inhibitors, hydralazine)
Beta-blockers
Ethanol
Tricyclic antidepressants (particularly amitriptyline, trimipramine, amoxapine)
Phenothiazines (particularly chlorpromazine, thioridazine, thiothixene)
Levodopa and dopamine agonists
Monoamine oxidase inhibitors

cause orthostatic hypotension are listed in Table 3.11. Orthostatic hypotension is usually worse early in the morning on rising from bed, or when getting out of a chair quickly. Elderly patients are well advised to perform simple leg exercises in the supine posture and to sit up slowly when getting out of bed. Other measures that may help include the reverse Trendelenburg position of the bed (using wooden or concrete blocks), a cautious increase of salt intake and fludrocortisone at a dose of 100–300 µg once daily. Blood pressure must be monitored carefully and particular caution is advised with fludrocortisone, which may result in peripheral oedema, unmasking of cardiac failure and significant hypokalaemia. Sometimes, compression stockings may help by improving venous return in the standing posture. However, it is important to demonstrate this benefit and the patient's ability to apply and remove the stockings before recommending their use.

Vasovagal syncope is usually diagnosed from the history, but where doubt exists and episodes are frequent, symptoms may be reproduced by prolonged head-up tilt table testing (although the significance of this procedure is controversial). In cases of recurrent vasovagal syncope or presyncope, the measures appropriate for orthostatic hypotension should be adopted and prolonged standing avoided. Sometimes, symptoms occur predictably within 90 minutes of a full meal, so-called **postprandial hypotension**. This is thought to be mediated by insulin or gut hormone release with food (since it responds to subcutaneous somatostatin), and may be alleviated by smaller meals more frequently and caffeine after eating.

In 1–2% of cases, syncope results from **carotid sinus syndrome**, where patients experience dizziness or actual syncope resulting from pressure on or stretching of the carotid sinus. This leads to sinus arrest lasting >3 seconds and/or a fall in systolic blood pressure >50 mmHg, resulting in cerebral hypoperfusion and syncope. Symptoms may be reproduced by gentle carotid massage, with simultaneous continuous non-invasive blood pressure (using Finapres servoplethysmography) and ECG readout, provided there is no contraindication to the manoeuvre, such as carotid stenosis, previous TIA or stroke. Those with reproducible cardio-inhibition usually improve with a **dual chamber permanent pacemaker**. There is no proven effective, safe, well-tolerated therapy for the vasodepressor variety of carotid sinus syndrome, but the non-pharmacological measures adopted for management of symptomatic orthostatic hypotension are appropriate.

Ageing is associated with some blunting of the normal equilibrium-maintaining mechanisms (vestibular, visual, proprioceptive and neuromuscular), so-called **presbystasis**, which may cause mild vertigo. More commonly, **vertigo** is the result of abnormal movement of calcium carbonate crystals (otoconia) from the saccule into the posterior semicircular canal, causing inappropriate stimulation of hair cells on head movement. This results in so-called **benign positional vertigo**, which is reproduced by passive head down tilt (45 degrees) with the head rotated by 45 degrees. Vertigo may also result from a variety of other causes (Table 3.12). **Ménière's disease** is overdiagnosed as the cause of vertigo in many elderly people. Ménière's disease is an uncommon condition and is characterized by recurrent attacks of vertigo over months or years, associated with tinnitus or deafness and severe nausea/vomiting. Treatment with so-called '**labyrinthine sedatives**' (**betahistine, cinnarizine,**

Table 3.12 Causes of vertigo in old age

Benign positional vertigo
Acute labyrinthine infections (usually viral)
Ménière's disease
Transient ischaemic attacks
Small vessel disease of the labyrinth (e.g. diabetes mellitus)
Hypothyroidism
Degenerative cervical spondarthritis

Table 3.13   Drug causes of vertigo

High doses/plasma levels of:
  Aminoglycosides
  Frusemide, bumetanide
  Ethanol
  Broad-spectrum anticonvulsants
  Quinine
  Non-neuroleptic hypnosedatives (e.g. benzodiazepines)

prochlorperazine, antihistamines) may be helpful in the short term (i.e. days to weeks) for severe vertigo, but long-term use is not advisable because of the risk of side-effects. 'Vestibular rehabilitation' (repetitive exercises that provoke vertigo, whilst teaching the patient to develop existing visual and proprioceptive compensatory mechanisms) may be helpful in younger patients with labyrinthine vertigo, but its practical value in elderly patients is uncertain. **Drugs may cause severe vertigo** (Table 3.13) and should not be forgotten in the differential diagnosis.

FURTHER READING

Anonymous. Managing carotid stenosis. *Drug Ther Bull* 1998; 36:9–12.
Anonymous. Management soon after a stroke. *Drug Ther Bull* 1998; 36:51–54.
Bakheit AMO, McLellan DLL. Parkinson's disease and other forms of Parkinsonism. In: CJ Goodwill, MA Chamberlain, C Evans (eds). *Rehabilitation of the Physically Disabled Adult*, 2nd edn. Stanley Thornes Publishers, Cheltenham, pp 457–476.
Downton JH. *Falls in the Elderly.* Edward Arnold, London, 1993.
Kapoor WN. Syncope in older persons. *J Am Geriatr Soc* 1994; 42:426–436.
Kenny RA (ed). *Syncope in the Older Patient.* Chapman & Hall Medical, London, 1996.
Quinn N. Drug treatment of Parkinson's disease. *Br Med J* 1995; 310:575–579.
Tallis R. *Epilepsy in the Elderly.* Martin Dunitz, London, 1996.
Warlow CP, Dennis MS, van Gijn J et al. A practical approach to the management of stroke patients. In: *Stroke: A Practical Guide to Management.* Blackwell Science, Oxford, 1996, pp 360–384.

Chapter 4

Respiratory Disorders

4.1 CHRONIC OBSTRUCTIVE PULMONARY DISEASE (COPD)

4.1.1 Assessment and Treatment of Stable COPD

The term 'chronic obstructive pulmonary disease' (COPD) encompasses those disorders characterized by chronic airflow limitation and certain typical features, including chronic bronchitis (with associated mucus hypersecretion), emphysema (with associated destruction of alveolar tissue) and asthma (with reversibility of airflow obstruction that improves with inhaled and/or oral corticosteroids). Most cases of COPD result from longstanding cigarette smoking, but it should be remembered that approximately half of all elderly asthmatics experience symptoms for the first time after age 65. The prevalence of asthma is estimated to be between 6.5% and 17% and is likely to increase as the proportion of elderly people in the general population rises. Asthma in old age is associated with greater morbidity and mortality than in younger age groups: approximately half of all asthma deaths occur in persons aged 65–84 years. This is thought to be the result of under-diagnosis and under-treatment, as well as a high rate of poor drug compliance (20–40%). Another possible reason is the under-use of inhaled corticosteroids, the mainstay of asthma treatment, in elderly asthmatics. Elderly people who are chronically dyspnoeic may be misdiagnosed with respiratory infection or cardiac failure and vice versa and given incorrect therapy, unless investigated appropriately at first presentation. The severity of COPD may be underestimated and undertreated in older people, who tend to be less physically active than younger people. Even when elderly patients are prescribed appropriate therapy for COPD, many will either fail to comply adequately or will have difficulty taking the medication, often because of poor technique with inhaler devices.

Accurate diagnosis with spirometry is the first step to effective therapy at all ages. Spirometry in elderly people, particularly frailer people, may present difficulties using conventional equipment that requires dexterity, timing and at least moderate upper limb strength. In recent years, light-weight, hand-held digital spirometry devices have considerably simplified pulmonary function testing, particularly for older patients, so that accurate diagnoses are now easily obtainable in most patients. However, these devices need regular servicing to maintain accurate readings. The diagnosis of COPD is defined by a forced expiratory volume in 1 second (FEV_1) <80% predicted and FEV_1 forced vital capacity (FVC) ratio <70%. Spirometry is preferable to peak expiratory flow rates, which have to be repeated several times over the space of one week to exclude variability in readings. The next step is grading patients' symptoms as mild (60–80% of predicted FEV_1), moderate (40–60%) or severe (<40%). All patients should be encouraged to quit smoking regardless of severity of symptoms. Sustained abstinence may be helped by taking part in an active cessation programme and use of nicotine replacement therapy. There is no reason why many elderly people should not take part in such programmes.

All patients with moderate or severe symptoms should have a trial of oral corticosteroids (e.g. prednisolone 30 mg daily for 2 weeks only) to look for significant reversibility of airflow limitation. Significant reversibility to corticosteroids is said to be present when there is an improvement of 15% and 200 ml or more in FEV_1 from baseline. Typically, the response is greater in cases of pure asthma, but more important is the detection of significant reversibility rather than putting a specific diagnostic label on the type of COPD. Objective reversibility of airflow obstruction with inhaled bronchodilators (e.g. salbutamol 2.5 mg by nebulizer) or oral corticosteroids is seen in 10–20% of cases, and these patients will usually benefit from long-term inhaled corticosteroids. It is important that all patients with significant reversibility from corticosteroids should understand the difference between corticosteroid preventive therapy and bronchodilator therapy for immediate symptom relief if compliance is to be maintained and exacerbations of COPD are to be treated appropriately.

Recommended therapy for patients with mild, moderate or severe COPD is detailed in Table 4.1. Particular caution is advisable when treating elderly COPD patients with oral bronchodilators, i.e. theophylline and long-acting beta-2 agonists. Theophylline should be given as a modified-release preparation, initially in low dosage (outside the emergency situation) since unmodified theophylline is absorbed rapidly and may induce side-effects such as tachyarrhythmias. Theophylline may also cause nausea, vomiting, hypokalaemia and convulsions, and toxic plasma levels may occur in patients treated concurrently with erythromycin, clarithromycin and ciprofloxacin. Elderly patients are particularly prone to tremor with long-acting beta-2 agonists, and special caution should be observed in those with coexistent arrhythmias and angina pectoris. Depressive illness is common in patients with moderate-to-severe COPD and should be specifically sought and treated.

A number of non-pharmacological measures may be beneficial also. Patients should exercise regularly in order to maximize aerobic fitness and optimize lung function. Obesity or malnutrition should be corrected

Table 4.1   Treatment of chronic obstructive pulmonary disease (COPD)

Severity of COPD	FEV_1 (% predicted)	Recommended treatment
Mild	60–80%	Short-acting beta-2 agonist or anticholinergic as required (e.g. salbutamol 200 µg or ipratropium bromide 40 µg, i.e. 2 puffs of MDI)
Moderate	40–60%	Regular therapy with beta-2 agonist or anticholinergic or both (e.g. 2 puffs of MDI q.i.d.) Consider a steroid trial (see text)
Severe	<40%	Regular therapy with beta-2 agonist *and* anticholinergic (2 puffs of MDI q.i.d.), *plus* Steroid trial in *all* patients and regular inhaled steroid (e.g. beclomethasone 200–400 µg b.i.d.) for all those with significant positive response (see text), *plus* Consider additional therapy, such as inhaled long-acting beta-2 agonist (e.g. salmeterol 50–100 µg b.i.d.) or modified-release theophylline 175–250 mg b.i.d.*

*Theophylline/aminophyllline is of limited value.
MDI, metered dose inhaler; b.i.d., twice daily; q.i.d., four times daily.
Adapted from British Thoracic Society: Guidelines for the management of chronic obstructive pulmonary disease. *Thorax* 1997; 52(Suppl 5): S1–S28, with permission from the BMJ Publishing Group.

where possible, since both conditions reduce ventilatory efficiency. Formal pulmonary rehabilitation programmes and long-term home oxygen therapy (LTOT) may be helpful for some selected patients with moderate or severe COPD (see below). Assessment of the elderly COPD patient's home circumstances by the occupational therapist is recommended, not just in relation to facilities for home nebulizer or LTOT, but also to look at ways of limiting physical effort in activities of daily living. Annual influenza vaccination is recommended for all elderly patients with moderate or severe COPD.

COPD in older people may be undertreated because of failure to adhere to recommended treatment guidelines on bronchodilator therapy for adults, such as those issued in the UK by the British Thoracic Society (see Table 4.1) and prescription of inhaler devices that may be suitable for younger, more able-bodied asthmatics, but inappropriate for elderly patients. The key to optimal management of COPD in elderly patients is tailoring the appropriate method of inhaled bronchodilator delivery to the patient's needs, using one of the wide variety of inhaler devices now available. For preventive therapy, a metered dose inhaler (MDI, i.e. aerosol type canister) alone or with a large volume spacer (LVS, e.g. Volumatic or Nebuhaler) is suitable in fit elderly patients. For less fit patients, MDI + LVS or a breath-actuated MDI may be more suitable. For relief of acute symptoms, MDI + LVS or breath-actuated MDI drug delivery is recommended, or nebulizer if acute exacerbations are frequent and severe. Dry powder devices are generally less suitable for older patients. Those patients with poor hand function or inability to coordinate deep inspiration with aerosol delivery may benefit from devices to place over the MDIs to facilitate operation (e.g. Haleraid). Examples of these inhaler devices are displayed in Figures 4.1 to 4.4. Nebulizers have become considerably more portable, more compact and less expensive in recent years, making them particularly suitable for those elderly patients who are unable to manage hand-held inhalers or spacer devices.

4.1.2 Infective Exacerbations of COPD

When patients present with exacerbations of previously stable COPD, this is commonly due to infection, failed treatment compliance,

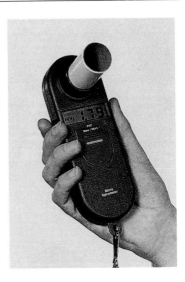

Figure 4.1 Portable digital spirometer. Reproduced by permission of Micro Medical Ltd, Rochester, Kent, UK

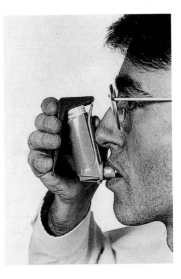

Figure 4.2 Device (Haleraid™) for patients with impaired hand function needing to use metered dose inhalers. Reproduced by permission of Allen & Hanburys, Uxbridge, UK

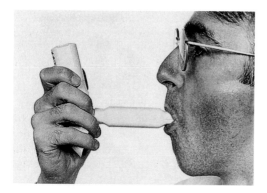

Figure 4.3 Breath-actuated metered dose inhaler with mini-spacer device (Easi-Breathe™). Reproduced by permission of Norton Healthcare Ltd, Harlow, Essex, UK

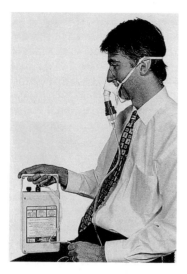

Figure 4.4 Rechargeable portable nebulizer. Reproduced by permission of DeVilbiss Medequip Ltd, Wollaston, West Midlands, UK

inadequate or inappropriate treatment. Increased sputum volume and purulence usually indicate infection and if associated with increased dyspnoea, an antibiotic is usually indicated. Corticosteroids should **not** be added to the therapy regimen **unless**

(i)   The patient is already on oral corticosteroids.
(ii) Significant reversibility has been shown to occur with previous steroid trial.
(iii) Airflow limitation fails to improve with increased doses of bronchodilators.
(iv) The patient is presenting with COPD for the first time.

Appropriate corticosteroid therapy is prednisolone 30 mg daily (or hydrocortisone 100 mg twice daily if oral therapy not suitable). This dose should be maintained for 7–14 days, depending on severity of the episode and the response to treatment. High dose beta-2 agonist therapy (10–20 puffs) via large volume spacer may be helpful in the short term. If this is not effective, temporary use of a nebulizer may be helpful for home management, particularly where there is doubt about the patient's current ability to manage other inhaler devices. If patients are unable to cope at home, are cyanosed, drowsy, severely breathless, have comorbid illnesses or usually require LTOT, hospital management is usually necessary. These patients usually require nebulized beta-2 agonist and ipratropium bromide in combination and supplemental oxygen (starting with 24–28% by mask or 2 l/min by nasal cannulae) adjusted according to arterial blood gas measurement. The role of intravenous aminophylline in acute exacerbations of COPD is increasingly doubtful. Many respiratory physicians reserve aminophylline infusion for patients with respiratory failure in whom doxapram is poorly tolerated or contraindicated.

The three most likely pathogens in patients with acute infective exacerbations of COPD are *Haemophilus influenzae*, *Streptococcus pneumoniae* and *Moraxella catarrhalis*. Atypical pathogens like *Mycoplasma pneumoniae*, *Chlamydia pneumoniae* and *Legionella pneumophila* are relatively uncommon. Sputum culture and antibiotic sensitivity should always be sought in more severe exacerbations of COPD to guide rational antibiotic therapy. Oral antibiotics are usually adequate except in severe cases. **Amoxycillin** or **tetracycline** (if penicillin-allergic) are the first choice drugs. If patients fail to respond to these, suitable second-line therapy is a broad-spectrum cephalosporin (e.g. **cefuroxime**) or **clarithromycin** (see section 4.2). Respiratory failure with infective COPD exacerbation may call for ventilatory support (see section 4.4).

4.2 TREATMENT AND PREVENTION OF PNEUMONIA

Pneumonia is the fifth leading cause of death in the USA and is the major infectious disease cause of morbidity and mortality in elderly people. The incidence of pneumonia in the general elderly US population is 20–40/1000/year, i.e. 5–10 times that in young adults. Among frail elderly people living in nursing and residential homes, the incidence is as high as 250/1000/year. There are several reasons why pneumonia is more common in elderly people, some age-related, others related to comorbid illness.

Age-related factors include:

(i)   High incidence of occult aspiration coupled with epiglottic or oesophageal dysfunction and less efficient cough reflex.
(ii) Less efficient bronchial mucociliary function.
(iii) Increased rate of oropharyngeal colonization with pathogenic organisms.
(iv) Reduced lymphocyte-mediated immunity in the bronchial tree.

Comorbidity-related factors include:

(i)   Reduced alveolar macrophage function in diabetes mellitus, chronic renal failure and malnutrition.
(ii) Concurrent cardiac failure associated with more severe infections.
(iii) Frail elderly people living in nursing homes prone to contracting virally mediated respiratory tract infections from one another, predisposing to secondary bacterial pneumonia.

It may be difficult to diagnose pneumonia clinically in some older patients because of absence of clinical symptoms and signs commonly seen in younger patients, such as productive cough, fever, focal pulmonary signs (basal inspiratory crackles may be found in some normal, healthy elderly people) and leucocytosis. Instead, elderly patients may present with lethargy, non-specific malaise, 'off-legs', 'taken-to-bed' or acute confusion, without overt respiratory symptoms. Even when pulmonary consolidation is detected radiologically, it is often not possible to isolate the pathogen because of failure to produce sputum, particularly in frail elderly patients. Unfortunately, there is no easy way to overcome this obstacle to microbiological detection of pathogens, although chest physiotherapy and inhaled nebulized 3%

saline may help expectoration. Gram stain detection of intracellular organisms before laboratory culture may be a valuable early indication of the likely pathogen. Even with sufficient sputum collection, however, cultures have a 30–40% pathogen detection rate. Therefore, in sick elderly patients with suspected pneumonia who are unable to expectorate **blood cultures should always be done**. Positive blood cultures are found in 15–25% of patients with pneumococcal pneumonia.

In elderly patients with pneumonia, antibiotic therapy often needs to be empirical, and initiation of therapy should not be delayed whilst microbiological detection of the pathogen is awaited. The choice of antibiotic therapy depends on several factors, such as known concurrent or previous respiratory disease, immune status and whether infection developed whilst in the community, in hospital or in long-term care facilities. Other circumstances, like aspiration and concurrent influenza, also influence the choice of drug. Details of empirical antibiotic choice are listed in Table 4.2. Resistance of *Haemophilus influenzae* to amoxycillin and ampicillin in the UK is increasing, currently 10% of isolates. Therefore, a cephalosporin (e.g cefuroxime) or coamoxiclav or one of the newer macrolides (e.g. clarithromycin or azithromycin) should be introduced when patients fail to respond to initial empiric therapy with amoxycillin. The third major pathogenic cause of infective exacerbation of COPD is *Moraxella catarrhalis* which is usually sensitive to coamoxiclav, cefuroxime and tetracycline. Gram-negative Enterobacteriaceae are the significant pathogens in many frail elderly nursing home residents with pneumonia and broad-spectrum empiric therapy with cefuroxime or ciprofloxacin is recommended in severe cases or when patients fail to respond to initial amoxycillin therapy.

Atypical pneumonia is not uncommon in elderly people. Recent studies have implicated *Chlamydia pneumoniae* in 5–10% of cases of infective exacerbation of COPD. Viruses are responsible for 10–15% of community-acquired lower respiratory tract infections, usually influenza (see below), respiratory syncytial virus and rhinovirus, which often occur in epidemics and may be complicated by secondary bacterial infection. Pneumonia due to *Mycoplasma pneumoniae* (5%) is uncommon in community-dwelling elderly people, but should be considered during epidemics and when beta-lactam antibiotic therapy is ineffective.

Table 4.2 Antibiotic therapy for pneumonia

Clinical situation	Likely organisms	Antibiotic
Primary pneumonia (previously healthy)	*Pneumococcus*	Amoxycillin 500 mg t.i.d. p.o. or IV
Known COPD	*Pneumococcus, Haemophilus influenzae*	Amoxycillin 500 mg t.i.d. p.o./IV or, if penicillin allergy, tetracycline 250–500 mg q.i.d. or cefuroxime 250 mg b.i.d. p.o. or 750 mg t.i.d. IV
Aspiration pneumonia	*Pneumococcus, Klebsiella pneumoniae*, anaerobic streptococci	Amoxycillin 500 mg t.i.d. IV + metronidazole 500 mg t.i.d. IV
Infective exacerbation of bronchiectasis	*Pneumococcus, Haemophilus influenzae, Pseudomonas*	As for infective COPD exacerbation Ciprofloxacin 500 mg b.i.d. p.o. or IV or ceftazidime 1 g t.i.d. IV
Influenza epidemic*	*Pneumococcu, Haemophilus influenzae, Staphylococcus aureus*	Coamoxiclav 375 mg t.i.d. p.o. or cefuroxime 250 mg b.i.d. or clarithromycin 250 mg b.i.d.
Atypical pneumonia†	*Mycoplasma pneumoniae, Chlamydia pneumoniae, Legionella pneumophila*	Erythromycin 0.5–1 g b.i.d. IV or 250–500 mg q.i.d. p.o. Add rifampicin 600 mg b.i.d. if *Legionella* infection confirmed
Severe pneumonia	Any organism but no time to identify	Cefotaxime 1–2 g t.i.d. + erythromycin 1 g q.i.d. IV

In general, treatment is given for 7–10 days. In frail elderly persons living in long-term care facilities, treatment duration may need to be extended to 14–21 days.

*In severely ill patients, antibiotic therapy should be given intravenously at appropriate doses alone or in combination with flucloxacillin.
†Treat for at least 10–14 days.
IV, intravenously; p.o., by mouth; b.i.d., twice daily; t.i.d., three times daily; q.i.d., four times daily.

Macrolides (e.g. erythromycin) are usually effective in confirmed cases of *Mycoplasma* and *Chlamydial* infection. Diagnosis of atypical pneumonia is confirmed by positive paired plasma serological tests showing rising specific antibody titres, but empiric antibiotic therapy should always be started before serological diagnosis.

Table 4.3 Recommendations for pneumococcal vaccination

Persons at increased risk of pneumococcal disease:
  (i)   Chronic cardiac or pulmonary disease
  (ii)   Chronic renal failure or nephrotic syndrome
  (iii) Chronic liver disease
  (iv)   Asplenism
  (v)   Diabetes mellitus
  (vi)   Chronic immunodeficient or immunosuppressed states

Pneumococcal polysaccharide vaccine affords protection against the 23 most prevalent pneumococcal serotypes of *Streptococcus pneumoniae*. The World Health Organization and the Immunization Practices Committee in the United States recommend pneumococcal vaccine for all persons over 65. The 3-year protective efficacy in those aged over 65 is 60–70%, although it falls to 46% in those aged over 85 years. Despite this, the cost–benefit balance is in favour of widespread use of the vaccine in elderly people. If resources limit its use, those at greatest risk from invasive pneumococcal disease should be targeted for vaccination (Table 4.3). Splenectomized persons at all ages are at high risk of pneumococcal septicaemia, and should have additional *Haemophilus influenzae* type b vaccine, with follow-up antibody titre measurement to ensure responses to immunization. The dose of pneumococcal vaccine is 0.5 ml by intramuscular injection.

4.3 INFLUENZA IN OLD AGE

Influenza occurs in winter epidemics and although the virus isolation rate in elderly people is similar to that in younger people, elderly people suffer much higher rates of morbidity and mortality. This is particularly true in elderly people with chronic diseases, such as COPD, cardiac failure, diabetes mellitus and chronic renal failure, and there is a direct relationship between the number of concurrent chronic diseases and influenza-related hospitalization and mortality rate. About one in four elderly people with influenza develops complications, particularly bronchitis and pneumonia, which may be due to primary influenzal infection or secondary bacterial infection. The most important secondary bacterial pathogens are *Streptococcus pneumoniae* and *Staphylococcus aureus*. The incidence of staphylococcal pneumonia increases two to three times during influenza epidemics and carries a particularly high mortality rate (20–30%).

Influenza is preventable in most elderly people with influenza immunization (see below). Once symptoms are noted, usually in the midst of a confirmed epidemic, elderly people should be treated with **amantadine**, analgesics, antipyretics and increased fluids (see Table 4.4). Amantadine reduces illness severity in most cases of influenza A, but has no efficacy in influenza B. It prevents influenza in about half of elderly people at risk, and may have a particularly important role during epidemics between the time of immunization and establishment of active immunity, i.e. 2–3 weeks, in those at high risk from the infection and in elderly people living in long-term care facilities. Amantadine may cause dizziness, confusion, insomnia and seizures in epileptic patients. A new derivative of amantadine, rimantadine, is believed to cause fewer side-effects, but is not yet widely available. Amantadine is effective if commenced within 48 hours of onset of influenza symptoms, but thereafter, it has little value.

With accurate characterization of the changes in haemagglutinins and raminidase enzymes on the influenza virus cell surface, with each

Table 4.4   Influenza treatment and prevention in older people

---

(A) Treatment
Amantadine 100 mg daily within 48 hours of onset of symptoms for 4–5 days
Symptomatic treatment of fever, myalgia, cough, dehydration.

(B) Prevention before epidemic
Intramuscular injection of 0.5 ml of inactivated influenza vaccine for those with:
- Chronic respiratory disease
- Chronic heart disease
- Chronic renal or liver failure
- Diabetes mellitus
- Immunosuppression due to disease or treatment; and those patients
- Living in nursing homes, residential homes or other long-stay care facilities where rapid spread is likely to follow introduction of infection.

(C) Prevention during epidemic
Intramuscular injection of 0.5 ml of inactivated influenza vaccine *plus* amantadine 100 mg daily for 2–3 weeks until active immunity established

---

influenza epidemic it is possible to prepare an effective live, attenuated virus vaccine. An effective influenza prevention programme also depends on predicting the time of an epidemic, identifying at-risk elderly people and giving the vaccine in a systematic way. At present, epidemic prediction and provision of effective vaccine is satisfactory in most Western countries. Effective immunization programmes reduce the influenzal complication rate by 60–90%, influenza-related hospital admissions by 50–100% and influenza-related mortality by 60–100%. Immunization should take place in mid-autumn so that full immunity with optimal levels of protective antibodies can develop before the peak prevalence winter months. To prevent influenza outbreaks in long-term care facilities, it is estimated that there must be a vaccine uptake rate in excess of 80%. Influenza vaccine is generally well tolerated by the majority of frail elderly people. In some, it may cause mild influenza-like symptoms, which usually disappear after 48 hours, and which respond to simple analgesics and antipyretics. The only important contraindication to influenza vaccine is allergy to egg yolk protein, since the vaccine is prepared in chick egg yolk sacs.

Secondary bacterial pneumonia is the major cause of death from influenza. The usual pathogens (*Streptococcus pneumoniae*, *Haemophilus influenzae*) are identified from sputum cultures, but *Staphylococcus aureus* is detected alone or in combination with another pathogen in 20–25% of cases. Therefore, empiric antibiotic therapy in these gravely ill patients should be effective against *Streptococcus pneumoniae*, *Haemophilus influenzae* and *Staphylococcus aureus*. Suitable choices are **cefuroxime**, **clarithromycin** or **coamoxiclav**, **alone or in combination with flucloxacillin**. In hospitals or long-term care facilities, methicillin-resistant *Staphylococcus aureus* (MRSA) may be the infecting organism. Here, intravenous **vancomycin** may be required. Where this is a significant possibility, vancomycin should be started in severely ill patients, whilst culture results are awaited.

4.4 RESPIRATORY FAILURE

Acute respiratory failure in old age most commonly results from exacerbations of COPD. It may occur from a variety of other causes, in particular acute-on-chronic congestive cardiac failure, pulmonary embolism, pneumothorax, systemic sepsis and drugs that suppress respiratory drive. Type I respiratory failure is defined by hypoxia ($PaO_2 < 8.0$ kPa) with normal or reduced $PaCO_2$, while type II respiratory failure is defined by hypoxia **plus** an increased $PaCO_2$, i.e. >5.3 kPa. Elderly patients with infective COPD exacerbations are particularly vulnerable to respiratory failure because of old age-related reduced respiratory muscle reserve leading to earlier respiratory muscle fatigue. This results in further impairment of gas exchange leading to further hypoxia and hypercapnia. All patients with respiratory failure require supplemental oxygen, which may be given by nasal cannulae, simple mask, Venturi mask or non-rebreathing mask. If these are ineffective or inappropriate (e.g. acute severe type II respiratory failure with deteriorating ventilatory drive), invasive mechanical ventilation may be necessary. Nasal cannulae and simple masks may deliver fractional inspired oxygen (FiO_2) concentrations of 24–40% at oxygen flow rates of 2–6 l/min. Venturi masks may deliver higher FiO_2 rates of 24–50% at oxygen flow rates of 2–15 l/min, but will not achieve FiO_2 rates higher than 50%. For FiO_2 rates of 50–100%, a non-breathing mask system is required. This has a reservoir bag and a one-way valve to prevent expiration into the oxygen reservoir, and needs to fit tightly over the face.

When arterial pH falls to <7.26, with rising $PaCO_2$ despite supportive therapy with supplemental oxygen, mechanical ventilatory support must be considered. The main factors that favour or discourage ventilatory support are listed in Table 4.5. Usually, endotracheal intubation and mechanical ventilation with **intermittent positive pressure ventilation (IPPV)** are required. However, elderly people tolerate IPPV less well than younger patients, and mortality rates of 25–30% can be expected. In recent years, it has become possible to mechanically ventilate some elderly patients non-invasively, using appropriate close-fitting (i.e. minimal air leak) nasal and face masks connected to small, portable pressure-cycled or volume-cycled ventilator machines, so-called **non-invasive intermittent positive pressure ventilation (NIPPV)**. These non-invasive ventilation techniques deliver higher alveolar oxygen concentrations, and have proven highly useful for the treatment of respiratory failure resulting from acute exacerbations of COPD. NIPPV aims to unload the fatiguing respiratory musculature, with correction of the acidosis (which reduces respiratory muscle contractility), thereby increasing ventilation. The technique involves oxygen delivery under continuous positive airways pressure (CPAP) by means of nasal or full face mask. NIPPV via full face mask is preferable, particularly during extreme dyspnoea. Caution must be taken to avoid barotrauma and skin pressure necrosis over the bridge of the nose, making continued ventilation impossible. Response to therapy is monitored with continuous digital pulse oximetry and regular arterial blood gas measurement to check that the acidosis is receding. The target is to reduce the $PaCO_2$ by approximately 1 kPa every 1–2 hours. Once the patient is stable from the point of view of arterial blood gases and pH, it is advisable to continue ventilation for several hours. Most patients require 6–10 hours of ventilation for 4–7 days, gradually reducing the time spent on the NIPPV as improvement occurs. NIPPV has been shown to lessen the number of patients requiring IPPV and duration of hospitalization. However, confused patients and those with copious respiratory secretions do not generally tolerate NIPPV well. This, and the fact that the necessary equipment and expertise are not as yet widely available in UK hospitals means that NIPPV has restricted application in elderly patients with respiratory failure.

Respiratory stimulants, such as **doxapram**, may help maintain ventilation for 24–36 hours until the underlying cause, usually pneumonia, is under control. It is suitable for patients with an arterial pH <7.26 and/or hypercapnia and hypoventilation. Confusion, agitation and seizures may occur with doxapram, usually at the higher dose range or in patients with seizure diathesis.

Table 4.5 The decision to institute ventilatory support with IPPV

(A) Factors in favour
- (i) A treatable cause of respiratory failure, e.g. pneumonia, drug overdose
- (ii) First episode of respiratory failure
- (iii) Good quality of life and activity

(B) Factors against
- (i) Documented severe chronic respiratory disease, unresponsive to treatment
- (ii) Major comorbid illnesses, such as cardiac failure, malignancy
- (iii) Poor quality of life

NB. Age and PCO_2 are **not** significant predictors of outcome with IPPV.

4.5 DOMICILIARY LONG-TERM OXYGEN THERAPY

Chronic hypoxia causes marked and sustained pulmonary vasoconstriction as well as polycythaemia by stimulation of erythropoietin release from the kidneys. Over time, the sustained increase of right ventricular afterload leads to right ventricular decompensation and eventually failure (cor pulmonale). Chronic systemic hypoxia also leads to cerebral hypoxia, which in turn may cause impaired memory and other neuropsychological dysfunction. Two large studies in the early 1980s, the Nocturnal Oxygen Therapy Trial in the USA and the Medical Research Council (MRC) Trial in the UK, clearly showed survival benefits from sustained oxygen therapy. They also showed a dose–response relationship between average number of hours of daily oxygen therapy and survival. In the MRC study, 5-year survival improved from 25% to 41% with 15 hours of oxygen therapy per day. Long-term oxygen therapy (LTOT) also resulted in less polycythaemia, retardation of progression of pulmonary hypertension and improved neuropsychological status. The UK indications for LTOT are summarized in Table 4.6. The patient's condition should be stable, ideally for 3 months or more, and other causes for impaired respiratory function treated vigorously, e.g. cardiac failure, respiratory infection, and patients should be on optimum therapy for COPD. Arterial blood gas measurements should be made on at least two occasions 3 weeks apart; otherwise LTOT tends to be prescribed inappropriately. The geriatric day hospital is a suitable setting for patient

Table 4.6 Guidelines for long-term oxygen therapy

Absolute indications in patients with COPD
$PaO_2 < 7.3$ kPa $\pm$ $PaCO_2 > 6$ kPa
$FEV_1 < 1.5$ litres; FVC < 2 litres
Measurements to be stable on 2 occasions at least 3 weeks apart after bronchodilator therapy

Relative indication in patients with COPD
PaO_2 7.3–8.0 kPa plus pulmonary hypertension, peripheral oedema or nocturnal hypoxaemia

Palliation benefit in non-COPD conditions, e.g. end-stage pulmonary fibrosis

Contraindicated in patients who continue to smoke
Risk of fire plus increased concentrations of carboxyhaemoglobin reduce effectiveness of LTOT

---

assessment, provided there is ready access to blood gas analysis. Arterial blood gas measurement should be checked before, during and after sustained oxygen flow at 2 l/min via nasal cannulae.

LTOT may be administered by oxygen cylinder or, more conveniently, with an oxygen concentrator. An oxygen concentrator functions as a molecular sieve, separating atmospheric oxygen from ambient air. Regular servicing is required to sustain sufficient oxygen concentrations. In the UK, oxygen concentrators are prescribed under the National Health Service, and are as cost-effective as oxygen cylinders. They weigh approximately 25 kg and may be attached to a fixed point, or may be mobile. The inspired oxygen flow should be titrated upwards until the patient achieves a $PaO_2 > 8.0$ kPa without an unacceptable rise in $PaCO_2$. For optimal survival rates, oxygen therapy should be given for 15 hours/day or more. In particular, nocturnal oxygen therapy is recommended, since PaO_2 is known to fall during sleep (particularly REM sleep). Domiciliary assessment of the patient may be useful to monitor LTOT response.

Disadvantages of LTOT in some patients include drowsiness/confusion after starting therapy if FiO_2 is too high (in type II respiratory failure), psychological dependency, reduced mobility and fire hazard (LTOT is contraindicated in smokers and oxygen sources should not be placed near direct heat sources). Good compliance may also be demanding for the patient: in males, LTOT does not appear to improve survival until after 500 days' therapy.

4.6 PULMONARY REHABILITATION

In recent years, many hospitals and respiratory disease clinics have developed pulmonary rehabilitation programmes. These are aimed at optimizing lung function, general fitness and well-being as well as survival in patients with a variety of chronic respiratory disorders, principally COPD. Pulmonary rehabilitation programmes apply to elderly patients as much as to younger patients, perhaps more so, given the reduced physiological reserve of older patients and the increased prevalence of comorbid medical conditions. Essentially, pulmonary rehabilitation emphasizes optimization of drug therapy, stopping smoking, chest physiotherapy, education and psychological support, increased aerobic fitness with exercise training, oxygen therapy where indicated, optimal nutrition, home care and social support for more severely handicapped patients. Stopping smoking in particular should be stressed even in old age, since this has been shown to help correct pulmonary function towards normal. Respiratory muscle training alone is of doubtful value.

Most rehabilitation programmes are hospital-based, but domiciliary programmes may be preferable to hospital programmes for elderly patients, not least because of the risk of nosocomial respiratory infection in this patient group. It is unclear whether pulmonary rehabilitation produces gains in patient survival, probably because of the heterogeneous patient groups and even more heterogeneous rehabilitation methods used in studies to date. They do, however, improve patient well-being and quality of life. To improve exercise capacity and general health status, rehabilitation programmes must include an exercise schedule and patients must be motivated to continue with the exercise training after completion of the programme if benefit is to be maintained.

FURTHER READING

British Thoracic Society. Guidelines for the management of community acquired pneumonia in adults admitted to hospital. *Br J Hosp Med* 1993; 49:346–350.

Brochard L, Manchebo J, Wysocki M et al. Noninvasive ventilation for acute exacerbations of chronic obstructive pulmonary disease. *N Engl J Med* 1995; 333:817–822 (plus accompanying editorial).

Connolly MJ (ed). *Respiratory Disease in the Elderly Patient*. Chapman & Hall Medical, London, 1996.

Lucas Y, Wang E, Gaiety GO et al. Meta-analysis of respiratory rehabilitation in chronic obstructive pulmonary disease. *Lancet* 1996; 348:1115–1119.

Medical Research Council Working Group. Long term domiciliary oxygen therapy in chronic hypoxic cor pulmonale complicating chronic bronchitis and emphysema. *Lancet* 1981; i:681–686.

Moxham J. Respiratory failure. In: DJ Weatherall, JGG Ledingham, DA Warrell (eds). *Oxford Textbook of Medicine*, 3rd edn. Oxford Medical Publications, 1996, pp 2901–2906.

Nocturnal Oxygen Therapy Trial Group. Continuous or nocturnal oxygen therapy in hypoxaemic chronic obstructive lung disease. *Ann Intern Med* 1980; 93:391–398.

Chapter 5

Psychiatric Disorders

5.1 DELIRIUM

Delirium is reported in 24–28% of elderly persons (i.e. over 65) admitted to hospital with acute illness. It is usually manifest as cognitive impairment with an altered and often fluctuating level of consciousness; the precise DSM-IV diagnostic criteria for delirium are listed in Table 5.1. The ageing brain is particularly susceptible to delirium, possibly as a result of age-related reduced central cholinergic tone and the fact that cholinergic neurones which mediate attention, memory and arousal are particularly sensitive to hypoxaemia. Delirium is a common, non-specific presentation of acute illness in elderly patients, and each case must be evaluated carefully to identify the underlying cause(s). Appropriate treatment of correctable causes of acute confusion usually restores the premorbid cognitive status. Delirium is not always fully reversible, however. Recent data show that one-quarter or more of elderly patients diagnosed with delirium during hospitalization with acute illnesses have persisting cognitive or attentional deficits 6 months after discharge. Delirium is also associated with an acute mortality rate of 20–30%. The most common causes of acute confusion in older people are infection (urinary, respiratory), drug intoxication or with-

Table 5.1 DSM-IV* diagnostic criteria for delirium

(A) Impaired consciousness with reduced ability to focus, sustain and shift attention.
(B) Altered cognitive or perceptual function that is not attributable to a pre-existing disorder such as dementia.
(C) Development over a short period of time (hours to days) and tendency to fluctuate throughout the course of the day.
(D) Evidence of underlying medical causative condition from clinical or laboratory findings.

*DSM-IV: *Diagnostic and Statistical Manual of Mental Disorders*, 4th edn, 1994 (American Psychiatric Association).

drawal (Table 5.2), metabolic disorders and acute cerebrovascular events.

Non-drug methods of managing acute confusion are listed in Table 5.3. Drug therapy for troublesome symptoms of acute confusion should only be used as a last resort, when non-drug methods have failed, and there is a risk of the patient injuring him/herself or others, or inadvertently impeding the administration of essential drug therapy (such as intravenous antibiotics). In these circumstances, the drug of choice is a high-potency neuroleptic, such as **haloperidol**. Haloperidol may be given orally, or intravenously or intramuscularly in extreme situations. A suitable initial dose of haloperidol is 0.5–1 mg in less severe cases, with dose repetition every 20–30 minutes until the patient is calm. A regular dose of 1–2 mg three times daily may then be started and after 48 hours the drug is gradually withdrawn at a daily rate of 25% of the maximum daily dose. Haloperidol is less cardiotoxic than phenothiazines, although it may cause marked sedation, Parkinsonism, postural hypotension and QT interval prolongation in higher doses. If Parkinsonism occurs as a side-effect of neuroleptic therapy in elderly, confused patients, it is not advisable to give anticholinergic drugs (e.g. benzhexol, benztropine, orphenidrine) to counteract this effect, since they are likely to worsen the confusional state. In patients with severe, refractory symptoms, cautious addition of **lorazepam**, with its reliable absorption,

Table 5.2 Common causes of drug-induced acute confusion

Sedatives	Levodopa, dopamine agonists
Neuroleptics	Corticosteroids
Tricyclic antidepressants	Non-steroidal anti-inflammatory drugs
Opioid analgesics	Hypotensive drugs
Anticholinergics	Diuretics
Anticonvulsants	Antihistamines

Table 5.3 Non-pharmacological management of acute confusion

Quiet, calm environment	Passive orientation to time, place, person
Good lighting, particularly at night	Prevent/treat constipation
Adequate hydration, nutrition	Avoid physical restraints (except in extreme situations)
Easy access to toilet, commode	

short half-life, absence of active metabolites and re
presence of liver disease may be helpful. The us
0.5 mg and it may be given by the intramuscular or
necessary. Doses may be repeated every hour until the patient is ~~~~
However, side-effects of lorazepam may be prohibitive in some patients,
e.g. marked sedation, disinhibition, increased risk of falling and respiratory depression in hypoxaemic patients. Lorazepam is particularly
suitable for treating acute alcohol or benzodiazepine withdrawal states.

The PRN (as required) use of neuroleptics and other tranquillizing drugs
for confused elderly patients carries the potential for inappropriate
indications (such as non-specific 'agitation') and inappropriate duration
of therapy. Similarly, the practice of PRN supplementation of a regular
dose regimen is to be avoided because of the likelihood of failing to
achieve the target effect and increasing the risk of adverse effects.

5.2 DRUG THERAPY IN DEMENTIA

In most dementing illnesses, the primary pathology is untreatable. In
cerebrovascular dementia, however, there is some evidence that control
of hypertension, stopping smoking and low-dose aspirin may significantly slow the rate of deterioration of cognitive performance. However,
abnormalities such as hypothyroidism, vitamin B_{12} deficiency, folate
deficiency and positive syphilis serology are usually incidental findings
in demented patients, and there is little evidence that treatment of these
conditions improves the cognitive status. Nevertheless, deficiency states
in dementia are associated with significant morbidity and therefore
should be treated. Improvement or cure of chronic cognitive impairment
has been described with shunt procedures in obstructive hydrocephalus,
burr-hole drainage of subdural collections, immunosuppression of
intracranial vasculitis, antimicrobial therapy of chronic meningitis and
surgical resection of focal benign intracranial tumours. Severe depression in elderly patients may cause a mild to moderate form of the
dementia syndrome that responds to antidepressant therapy. However,
the majority of demented patients who are depressed have an underlying
organic dementing illness.

ιere has been a recent re-emergence of interest in cholinomimetic drugs in Alzheimer's disease (AD), in particular, **tacrine** (tetrahydro-aminoacridine; Cognex) and **donepezil** (Aricept) and **rivastigmine**. Both tacrine and donepezil have been licensed for the treatment of AD and rivastigmine will probably be soon available in the UK. These acetylcholinesterase inhibitors appear to produce benefit in some mildly impaired patients by preservation of acetylcholine in the synaptic cleft with enhanced neurotransmission. Therefore, they depend on intact cholinergic neurones for efficacy. As AD advances with increasing loss of cholinergic cells, these drugs are likely to lose whatever effect they may have. Based on current evidence, **tacrine** confers, at best, modest benefit and any improvements of cognitive function are temporary (weeks–months). Tacrine commonly causes cholinergic side-effects that are prohibitive, e.g. nausea, vomiting, diarrhoea, sialorrhoea, and it is hepatotoxic. A recent evaluation of the efficacy data from high-dose tacrine (160 mg daily) concluded that the likelihood of patients tolerating the drug and having an apparent improvement was approximately 10%.

Donepezil, on the other hand, is reported to cause fewer cholinergic, gastrointestinal and hepatotoxic side-effects. It binds preferentially to acetylcholinesterase in the brain, having little effect on plasma butyryl-cholinesterase and cholinesterase in the myocardium and small intestine. Peak plasma levels occur 3–4 hours after dosing and its biological half-life is about 3 days. It is metabolized by the hepatic cytochrome P450 system, which results in several active metabolites. At present, there is one published randomized, double-blind, placebo-controlled study of donepezil in mild–moderately impaired AD patients in the literature, showing a small but significant and dose-related benefit in cognitive status from active treatment. The starting dose of donepezil is 5 mg daily, increasing after 1 month to a maximum of 10 mg daily, if necessary. Donepezil is generally well tolerated, although side-effects such as diarrhoea, nausea and vomiting, muscle cramps, fatigue and insomnia occur twice as frequently as with placebo. The results of further studies are awaited, but on the basis of current evidence, donepezil cannot be recommended for widespread use in AD.

Depression must be confidently excluded in order to diagnose dementia. However, depression is not uncommon in the early stages of dementia and should be aggressively treated. In demented patients, tricyclic antidepressants may worsen the cognition and overall level of functioning because of their anticholinergic properties. It is therefore advisable to try a non-tricyclic agent as first-line therapy, such as **fluoxetine**, **paroxetine**, **sertraline** or **citalopram** (selective serotonin reuptake inhibitors (SSRIs)—see section 5.3). An alternative is **moclobemide** (see below), a selective, reversible inhibitor of monoamine oxidase A (RIMA), which is safe and well tolerated in elderly demented patients. Elderly demented patients are often unable to articulate depressive symptoms, and depression may manifest as crying episodes, food refusal, sad facial expression, agitation or aggression. A high index of suspicion and a lower threshold for empirical therapy are appropriate in these circumstances. Similarly, patients may not complain of drug side-effects as clearly as cognitively normal depressed patients, so increased vigilance for adverse side-effects of antidepressant therapy is necessary.

Drug therapy for persistent agitation or aggressive behaviour in demented patients should be considered as a last resort, when non-drug methods such as appropriate environmental changes (e.g. providing adequate space to 'wander safely'), adequate ambient lighting, reorientation, reassurance and minimization of distracting stimuli have failed. Some important precepts should be followed when commencing continuous drug therapy (Table 5.4). **Neuroleptics** are widely prescribed for chronic aggression/agitation in elderly demented patients. Neuroleptics are superior to placebo, but no single neuroleptic is more effective than any other, **thioridazine** and **haloperidol** being the most widely used drugs in published studies. Haloperidol (0.5–5 mg daily in divided doses) is usually effective in both acute and chronic behaviour disorder.

Table 5.4 Principles of drug therapy for agitated/aggressive behaviour in dementia

---

(i) The precise aetiology of the problem must be defined and remediable causes treated (e.g. physical illness, depression, psychosis)
(ii) The nature and extent of the problem must be clearly but succinctly documented
(iii) Select a drug that will abolish the target symptom(s), with the least side-effects
(iv) Use the smallest dose of a drug to achieve the desired effect
(v) Titrate drug dose slowly against intensity of target symptoms and side-effects
(vi) Make a plan specifying the duration and gradual withdrawal of therapy, once the desired effect has been achieved.

However, the use of neuroleptics is often limited by their tendency to cause **extrapyramidal side-effects** (EPS; Parkinsonism, tardive dyskinesia, akathisia, dystonias), when taken for more than a few days. Anticholinergic drugs to counteract EPS are generally unsuitable in elderly confused patients, due to serious side-effects. There is also some evidence that cognitive decline may be hastened by neuroleptic therapy in demented patients, although it is unclear whether the poorer prognosis results from the drug therapy or from dementia compounded by delusional features. Use of neuroleptics is contraindicated in dementia with Lewy bodies (DLB), because of the risk of extreme neuroleptic sensitivity leading to severe EPS that may be fatal. The phenomenon is thought to be mediated by the combination of subclinical reduction in substantia nigral neurones coupled with a failure of upregulation of D2 receptors in the corpus striatum, when there is substrate depletion or receptor blockade. The clinical features of DLB include higher cortical deficit (often attentional and/or visuospatial before memory), fluctuation of cognitive symptoms and alertness, recurrent visual hallucinations (typically well formed and detailed) and features of Parkinsonism.

In recent years, 'atypical' neuroleptics have emerged, principally **risperidone**, **olanzapine** and **clozapine**. These are distinguished from 'typical' neuroleptics by having substantially **lower risk of EPS**, possibly through their major antagonistic effects on 5-hydroxytryptamine ($5HT_2$) receptors. Risperidone is as effective as haloperidol in schizophrenic psychosis, and experience with risperidone in elderly demented patients so far has shown it to be safe. It may be suitable for patients at high risk from EPS such as demented patients with Parkinson's disease and Parkinsonism associated with cerebrovascular disease. The recommended starting dose of risperidone is 0.25–0.5 mg twice daily, increasing to a maximum dose of 1–2 mg twice daily in elderly patients. Olanzapine is an alternative to risperidone, is also less likely to cause EPS and its once daily dosage may be an advantage in doubtful treatment compliance. However, experience with olanzapine in elderly demented patients is limited. Clozapine may be less suitable for elderly demented patients, in view of its significant anticholinergic effects at medium and higher doses, and the fact that it carries a 1–2% risk of severe leucopenia. Clozapine is currently licensed in the UK only for treatment of schizophrenic patients who are resistant to other neuroleptics.

Thioridazine is also widely used in elderly patients with chronic agitation/aggressive behaviour disorder. Thioridazine is a **'low-potency' neuroleptic**, i.e. its dopamine D2 receptor inhibition is relatively weak compared to **'high-potency' neuroleptics**, such as haloperidol, fluphenazine and trifluoperazine. Low potency neuroleptics also have greater anticholinergic side-effects and therefore are more sedating than high potency neuroleptics, which have greater antipsychotic efficacy. Thioridazine does not treat the organic confusional state itself, but may make the patient more manageable for several weeks and, like other neuroleptics, it may actually worsen cognitive function. Thioridazine has a half-life of 21 hours, and it and its active metabolite tend to accumulate when treatment is prolonged. This may result in a vicious cycle of increasing confusion and escalating thioridazine dose. Thioridazine also has powerful alpha-adrenergic blocking effects, increasing the risk of symptomatic orthostatic hypotension. For these reasons, thioridazine is unsuitable in many elderly frail patients, in whom **short-term, low-dose, high potency neuroleptic therapy** is generally preferable.

Depot neuroleptic therapy should be avoided in elderly patients because of the increased risk of major EPS. However, in rare circumstances where patients with severe psychotic or behavioural symptoms consistently refuse oral medication and in whom non-drug behaviour modification has failed, short-term intramuscular administration of a non-depot neuroleptic may be tried, but only where close monitoring of efficacy and side-effects is available. If there is a favourable response to a test dose of oral or intramuscular haloperidol, depot fluphenazine decanoate, at one-quarter of the starting dose in young psychotic patients, can be given, continued weekly or fortnightly, but aiming to discontinue after two or three doses.

Alternatives to neuroleptic drugs should be considered where troublesome neuroleptic EPS occur, where neuroleptics have not been effective or are contraindicated. Despite a lack of good quality research trial data, small-scale studies indicate that **trazodone** and **carbamazepine** may be beneficial, where neuroleptics are unsuitable. Trazodone has been reported to reduce agitation and improve mood in Alzheimer's disease at doses up to 300 mg daily. It tends to cause sedation, so is best given at night-time. It is less liable to cause anticholinergic or cardiotoxic side-effects than tricyclic antidepressants, but it can cause orthostatic hypotension. Carbamazepine, at doses up to 800 mg daily, has been reported to be effective in aggressive/violent patients with organic brain syndromes. It has also been shown to improve severe behaviour disorder in Alzheimer's disease patients resistant to neuroleptic therapy and appears to be particularly suitable in patients with impulsive, agitated or aggressive episodes. Treatment should be continued for 6–8 weeks and then withdrawn. Carbamazepine may cause sedation, cerebellar dysfunction, hyponatraemia and anticholinergic side-effects.

5.3   ANTIDEPRESSANT THERAPY IN OLD AGE

Elderly people are at greatest risk from depressive illness. About 15% of all elderly people at any one time have significant depressive symptoms, and 1–4% have major depression that requires treatment. However, the diagnosis of major depression in old age may be less clearcut than in younger people. This is because major depressive somatic symptoms in older people such as weight loss, anorexia, altered sleep pattern and cognitive impairment may be caused by disorders other than depression. Also, depressive symptoms occurring in the context of some other major illness may be masked, making diagnosis of depression less clearcut. However, the core symptoms of depression in old age are fundamentally similar to those in younger people, and the risk of suicide is at least as high in older as in younger depressives. For example, in the UK, elderly people make up about 15% of the population, but account for 25% of all suicides. Certain clinical features occur more commonly in depressed old people, such as agitation, delusions, hypochondriasis, hallucinations and cognitive impairment. However, once major depression has been confidently diagnosed, the principles of treatment are similar regardless of age.

Tricyclic antidepressants are equally effective in older and younger age groups. However, elderly people are more susceptible to adverse side-effects with tricyclic drugs, i.e. sedation, dry mouth, constipation, urinary voiding problems, blurred vision, glaucoma, orthostatic hypotension, cardiac arrhythmias and hyponatraemia. Traditional tricyclics such as amitriptyline, imipramine and doxepin are particularly liable to cause adverse side-effects and should probably be avoided in elderly people nowadays, particularly with the wide range of effective and well tolerated alternative drugs that are available. Second-generation tricyclics, such as **lofepramine**, **desipramine** and **nortriptyline**, have fewer anticholinergic side-effects, are generally better tolerated and relatively safe following overdose in older people. Elderly patients require similar doses of antidepressant medication to younger patients for efficacy. The usual starting dose of lofepramine is 70 mg twice daily, which is increased to a maximum dose of 210 mg daily as required. A recommended checklist before tricyclic antidepressant treatment is illustrated in Table 5.5.

The treatment of depression in old age has been greatly helped by the introduction of SSRIs such as **fluoxetine**, **paroxetine**, **citalopram** and **sertraline**, which are now considered by many psychiatrists to be the first-line antidepressants in elderly people. SSRIs are considered particularly suitable for depressed patients with coexistent panic or major anxiety symptoms. These agents have the advantages of being non-sedating, better tolerated than tricyclic antidepressants and safe in overdose. Adverse side-effects, however, do occur with SSRIs and these may be problematic, i.e. transient anxiety/nervousness, insomnia, nausea/vomiting, abdominal discomfort, diarrhoea, headache and hyponatraemia. These side-effects usually resolve within a few weeks, but sexual dysfunction (reduced libido, anorgasmia) may be a continuing problem. Paroxetine also has clinically significant anticholinergic effects that are usually well tolerated in elderly people, but may worsen cognitive function in patients with AD. The SSRIs are competitive

Table 5.5 Pretreatment checklist of contraindications to tricyclic antidepressant therapy

(1) Glaucoma
(2) Prostatism
(3) Cardiac failure
(4) Orthostatic hypotension
(5) Cardiac conduction disorders including
    —bundle branch block
    —first degree heart bock
(6) Tachyarrhythmias
(7) Liver disease/altered liver function
(8) Severe constipation

inhibitors of the cytochrome P450 isoenzyme IID6, so that potentially serious adverse drug interactions from reduced drug metabolism may occur (e.g. warfarin, other antidepressants, anticonvulsants, beta-blockers, theophylline). Since SSRIs are highly protein-bound, they may also displace other highly protein-bound drugs (e.g. warfarin, phenytoin), causing toxicity. Particular caution should be observed with starting or discontinuing SSRIs in patients being treated with monoamine oxidase inhibitors (MAOIs), since SSRIs may enhance the effects of MAOIs and cause MAOI toxicity. The long half-lives of fluoxetine (2–3 days) and its active metabolite, norfluoxetine (7–9 days) facilitate once daily or alternate day dosage, a factor that may be helpful in patients with poor compliance. Paroxetine and sertraline have shorter half-lives, but once daily dosage is usually sufficient. Starting doses and maintenance doses are the same for paroxetine (20 mg daily) and fluoxetine (20 mg daily), which greatly simplifies the dose schedule. Paroxetine, in particular, is suitable in patients with compromised renal or hepatic function. The usual dose range for citalopram is 20–60 mg daily and for sertraline 50–100 mg daily. There is no good evidence that the combination of a tricyclic antidepressant and an SSRI is any more effective than either agent on its own. **Trazodone**, another antidepressant that works principally by inhibition of serotonin reuptake, is seldom used to treat depression in elderly people nowadays. It does not have anticholinergic properties, but it is highly sedative.

Another class of drugs that may be worth trying is the **reversible inhibitors of monoamine oxidase type A (RIMA). Moclobemide** is the first drug of this class to obtain a product licence. It is generally well tolerated in elderly people and it carries a much lower risk of tyramine-associated hypertensive reactions than with traditional MAOIs such as tranylcypromine and phenelzine. However, it is still recommended to limit the intake of tyramine-containing foods when taking moclobemide. Moclobemide should not be prescribed in patients taking levodopa (risk of hypertensive crisis) or opioid analgesics (risk of major central nervous system depression or agitation). It may also interact adversely with both tricyclics and SSRIs, and one should allow sufficient time between stopping one antidepressant and starting moclobemide (from 1 to 5 weeks, depending on the agent). Moclobemide is usually given in a starting dose of 150 mg twice daily, and adjusted up to a maximum dose of 600 mg daily.

Venlafaxine and **nefazodone** are new non-SSRI antidepressants that block both serotonin and noradrenaline reuptake. Experience with their use in elderly depressed patients so far is limited.

Electroconvulsive therapy (ECT) is still the treatment of choice in severely depressed patients who are at high risk of suicide or who have not responded to antidepressant drug therapy. Despite its 'bad press', ECT is usually effective and generally well tolerated by elderly patients. It is particularly suitable in patients

(i)   with delusions/psychosis or marked psychomotor slowing,
(ii) with high suicide risk,
(iii) with high risk of non-compliance with drug therapy,
(iv) who cannot tolerate or who have failed to respond to the various drug therapies.

Patients need to be off SSRIs (2 weeks for paroxetine, 6 weeks for fluoxetine) before starting ECT to minimize the risk of prolonged seizures during ECT. Its effect may be rapid, i.e. within days as opposed to weeks with antidepressant drugs. Bilateral, brief pulse ECT using a moderate suprathreshold stimulus is the method of choice in elderly patients. Seizure threshold must be carefully evaluated since the ECT dose often needs to be higher in elderly than in young patients, particularly elderly males. Unilateral non-dominant hemispheric treatment is the second choice method of ECT in older patients, and is recommended when patients suffer marked memory or other cognitive impairment following bilateral ECT treatment that endangers their personal safety. ECT is normally given twice or three times weekly until the patient's mood has improved and stabilized (usually 10–12 treatments). On completion of ECT, treatment with an antidepressant or lithium should be started to prevent relapse.

Lithium is another highly effective therapy for many elderly depressed patients, but like ECT, should only be prescribed with the supervision of a psychiatrist. The risk of lithium toxicity is greater in older than in younger patients, but this risk is minimized by careful adjustment of dosage and monitoring to maintain a plasma concentration of 0.4–0.7 mEq/l. Lithium is particularly helpful in preventing relapse of manic–depressive or recurrent depressive illness. Side-effects of lithium may be dose dependent or dose independent (Table 5.6). Important

Table 5.6   Side-effects of lithium therapy

(A) Dose-dependent:
Plasma level 1.5–3.0 mmol/l: ataxia, weakness, tremor, drowsiness, thirst, nausea, diarrhoea
Plasma level 3.0–5.0 mmol/l: dehydration, delirium, convulsions, spasticity, coma

(B) Dose-independent:
Hypothyroidism
Brady- and tachyarrhythmias
ECG T-wave flattening
Nephrogenic (pitressin-resistant) diabetes insipidus
Weight gain

---

potential adverse drug interactions with lithium include neuroleptics (EPS), thiazide diuretics (lithium toxicity) and non-steroidal anti-inflammatory drugs (lithium toxicity). Good renal function is required for safe lithium therapy and should be monitored, with thyroid function, on a regular basis. In relapsing or unresponsive major depression, lithium is often given to 'augment' other antidepressant drugs.

The natural history of untreated depressive illness in elderly people is that of a 2–4 year time course. Therefore, antidepressant therapy should be continued for 2 years and possibly longer. Even with continuous antidepressant therapy for 2 years, the relapse rate in elderly patients is approximately 30%.

5.4 TREATMENT OF PSYCHOTIC ILLNESS IN OLD AGE

Psychotic phenomena may occur in a variety of psychiatric conditions in old age, including dementia, depression, drug toxicity and withdrawal, alcoholism, schizophrenia and delusional disorder. In this section, drug therapy of the latter two primary psychotic disorders will be considered. An American study recently showed that schizophrenia accounts for about one-third of all elderly long-term inpatients in psychiatric hospitals and for one in every eight patients in nursing homes. In late-onset paranoid schizophrenia or 'late paraphrenia', elderly patients suffer from persecutory delusions often with hallucinations, but do not usually manifest the gross thought disorder and personality/affective disintegration seen in younger schizophrenics. In primary delusional disorder, patients have persistent false beliefs, such as being spied upon, cheated out of money or possessions, or being the victim of a conspiracy. Other psychiatric symptoms are often absent and intellectual and social function are usually well preserved.

Traditionally, the recommended treatment in late-onset paranoid schizophrenia and delusional disorder has been high potency neuroleptics, e.g. haloperidol, fluphenazine, trifluoperazine. However, elderly people are at high risk of EPS and tardive dyskinesia from these traditional neuroleptics. **Risperidone, olanzapine** and **sulpiride** are well tolerated in elderly psychotic patients, have a reduced risk of causing EPS and are therefore preferable to other neuroleptics. Tardive dyskinesia is noted in about 40% of elderly psychotic patients, for which there is no satisfactory treatment. If tardive dyskinesia becomes marked, the dose of neuroleptic should be reduced. Anticholinergic drugs (e.g. benzhexol, benztropine, orphenadrine) are not recommended for drug-related EPS in elderly people.

High potency neuroleptics should be avoided in **psychotic Parkinsonian patients**. Reduction of levodopa or dopamine agonist dosage is recommended first, but if psychosis persists, **risperidone** may be tried, starting at 0.5 mg twice daily. Dementia with Lewy bodies should be confidently excluded before starting risperidone because of the risk of severe EPS.

In the USA, legislation was introduced following the Omnibus Budget Reconciliation Act (OBRA, 1987) to guide the safe and appropriate use of antipsychotic drugs in long-term care facilities for elderly people who receive Medicare and Medicaid benefits. Essentially, the **OBRA guidelines** stipulate that patients should only receive antipsychotics for a specific agreed indication, that all attempts at dose reduction and drug discontinuation should be made, with suitable non-drug behavioural intervention unless clinically contraindicated. Specific indications for neuroleptics include psychotic disorders, delirium and dementia associated with psychotic or agitated behaviours that cause serious endangerment to self or others or reduce functional independence, and short-term treatment (i.e. 7 days) of hiccups, nausea, vomiting or pruritus. Table 5.7 lists the circumstances where antipsychotic drugs are inappro-

Table 5.7   Circumstances where antipsychotic drugs are inappropriate in old people

Wandering	Non-psychotic depression
Poor self-care	Insomnia
Restlessness	Unsociability
Impaired memory	Fidgeting
Anxiety	Nervousness
Indifference to surroundings	Uncooperativeness

Source: Omnibus Budget Reconciliation Act, 1987.

priate. Whilst antipsychotic prescription practices have improved in the United States following the introduction of OBRA guidelines, there is evidence of high rates of inappropriate neuroleptic prescription in UK nursing homes. A recent survey of 909 nursing home residents in Glasgow showed that approximately one-quarter were taking regular neuroleptics, in whom the drugs were clinically indicated in only 12% according to OBRA guidelines.

5.5   SLEEP DISORDERS IN OLD AGE

Insomnia is the commonest sleep disturbance in older people. Its prevalence rises steadily after age 50, and is a particular problem in long-term care facilities. Duration of sleep, depth of sleep and quantity of REM sleep decline as part of normal ageing. Sudden changes in sleep pattern are usually significant, and causes must be sought. Not uncommonly, there is underlying depression or anxiety, or a physical problem such as prostatism, constipation, angina pectoris or arthritis. Successful treatment of underlying problems usually cures the secondary insomnia. Older people often have personal habits that are not conducive to good 'sleep hygiene', like habitual intake of alcohol, caffeine or tobacco last thing at night. Inappropriate drugs may also be culpable, e.g. fluoxetine, corticosteroids or loop diuretics taken in the evening. High levels of noise and lighting in hospitals and institutional care facilities unfortunately still cause much sleep disruption in elderly patients, a problem that is all too often overlooked or disregarded as unimportant. A careful history will identify such causes, which may often be easily remedied without resorting to hypnotic drugs.

Hypnotic drugs should be used as a last resort for managing sleep disorder in old people, since adverse side-effects are more prevalent and serious than in younger patients, e.g. falls and confusion. Benzodiazepines with short plasma half-lives, such as **temazepam** (10–20 mg), **lormetazepam** (0.5–1 mg) and **lorazepam** (1–2 mg) are suitable drugs for elderly patients with insomnia. Alternatives are **zopiclone** (3.75–7.5 mg), a cyclopyrrolone that also acts on gamma-aminobutyric acid (GABA$_A$) receptors and **zolpidem** (5–10 mg), an imidazopyridine with similar mode of action to zopiclone. Hypnotic drugs should not be used for periods longer than 8 weeks, because of increased risk of dependence and side-effects, principally falls and confusion. For occasional use, **chlormethiazole** (1–2 capsules) is suitable. Use of antidepressants and neuroleptics as hypnotics is to be avoided. Similarly, sedative antihistamines should not be used to induce sleep because of their powerful anticholinergic effects and the rapid onset of drug tolerance, leading to dose escalation.

Sleep apnoea syndrome is said to affect approximately 4% of community-dwelling elderly people. It may be due to upper airway obstruction or brainstem control of respiratory drive, and the broken nocturnal sleep pattern may result in daytime fatigue and somnolence. Accurate diagnosis often requires polysomnographic assessment in a sleep laboratory. Its management depends on whether the cause is obstructive or central. In obstructive sleep apnoea, continuous positive airways pressure **(CPAP)** ventilation is often effective, when tolerated. In severely obese patients, steady weight reduction usually improves sleep apnoea. In all cases, it is important to avoid hypnotics, which tend to worsen sleep apnoea symptoms.

The symptom of **restless legs** (Ekbom's syndrome) increases in prevalence with ageing, causing painful leg cramps and a sensation of limb restlessness, particularly whilst in bed. Involuntary jerking movements of the legs may be so severe as to wake patients from their sleep. The aetiology is unknown, but a positive family history is recognized in about one-third of patients and restless legs may be associated with various underlying conditions, such as iron, folate or B$_{12}$ deficiency, peripheral neuropathy (particularly with uraemia, diabetes mellitus, rheumatoid arthritis) and certain drugs (e.g. neuroleptics, lithium, beta-blockers, tricyclic antidepressants, anticonvulsants, H$_2$-blockers).

The differential diagnosis includes vascular rest pain, muscle cramps, burning feet syndrome and akathisia. Physical signs are usually absent and neuromuscular investigation is usually negative (except where peripheral neuropathy is the underlying diagnosis). Underlying disorders should be treated where identified, and medications suspected of being causative should be stopped. For severe symptoms, a variety of agents may be tried, such as **levodopa**, **clonazepam** or **carbamazepine**. Quinine is not effective for restless legs.

5.6   MAJOR ANXIETY DISORDER IN OLD AGE

Severe anxiety in old age is usually a secondary manifestation of an underlying psychiatric illness, usually depression or dementia, or physical illness. It may also result from psychostimulants or sedative/alcohol withdrawal. Somatic symptoms of anxiety are often misinterpreted by both patients and their physicians as organic physical illness, which may engender further anxiety, particularly if extensive laboratory investigation is undertaken. Anxiety may occur with any severe acute illness, but this is usually appropriate to the clinical situation. Disabling anxiety that is not appropriate to the physical condition of the patient points to a primary psychiatric problem.

Because of the strong association of anxiety with underlying depression in old age, antidepressants are often given as first-line therapy for major anxiety even though depressive symptoms may not be prominent. Antidepressants are usually effective for suppression of anxiety that is secondary to underlying depression, obsessive compulsive disorder or recurrent panic disorder. **Selective serotonin reuptake inhibitors** are suitable as first-line therapy for major anxiety and panic attacks, although fluoxetine may itself sometimes **cause** anxiety symptoms. Tricyclic antidepressants may also be tried, but have greater risks of adverse side-effects, as mentioned earlier. **Benzodiazepines** are generally avoided for treatment of anxiety in old age because of their propensity to cause major adverse side-effects (e.g. falls, confusion) and dependency when taken over a long period. However, for short-term therapy, shorter-acting benzodiazepines may be helpful, e.g. lorazepam (0.5–3 mg twice daily) or oxazepam (5–20 mg three times daily). **Buspirone**, a $5HT_{1A}$-receptor antagonist, may be useful for longer-term suppression of anxiety. However, it may take 2–4 weeks to show a beneficial effect and benzodiazepines may be required in the interim. Buspirone has several attractive properties for older patients, i.e. it is non-sedative and non-addictive, does not cause withdrawal symptoms, is safe in overdose and carries little risk of adverse drug interaction (except for MAOIs). However, it may cause nausea, dizziness, headache and nervousness. The pharmacokinetics of buspirone are unchanged in old age and dosage in elderly patients is the same as in younger patients, i.e. 5 mg two to three times daily, increasing to a maximum of 45 mg daily in divided doses. Behavioural/relaxation therapy for major anxiety may be as beneficial in elderly as in young patients. Controlled breathing, muscle relaxation and Tai Chi Chuan physiotherapy techniques are effective in elderly patients and may be valuable adjuvants to pharmacotherapy in selected individuals.

5.7 IATROGENIC PSYCHOPATHOLOGY IN OLD AGE

Prescription drugs may cause or exacerbate confusional states (acute, subacute or chronic), mood disorder or anxiety. Table 5.2 lists the drugs known to cause or worsen confusion in old people. Drugs that may cause depression and anxiety are listed in Table 5.8.

Table 5.8 Drugs that may cause symptoms of depression and anxiety

(A) Depression	
Opioid analgesics	Benzodiazepines
NSAIDs	Ethanol
Antihypertensives, e.g.	Cytotoxic drugs, e.g.
lipophilic beta-blockers, e.g. propranolol	cisplatin
methyldopa	vincristine
clonidine	mitotane
Neuroleptics	Oral corticosteroids
H_2-blockers, e.g. cimetidine	Oestrogens
Thiazide diuretics	
(B) Anxiety	
Xanthines, e.g.	Fluoxetine
theophylline	Sympathomimetics, e.g.
aminophylline	phenylephrine
Beta-2 agonists	phenylpropanolamine
Withdrawal effects, e.g.	ephedrine
ethanol	
benzodiazepines	

FURTHER READING

Anonymous, Donepezil for Alzheimer's disease? *Drug Ther Bull* 1997; 35:75–76.

Davis KL. Tacrine. *Lancet* 1995; 345:625–630.

Katona CLE. New antidepressants in the elderly. In: C Holmes, R Howard (eds). *Advances in Old Age Psychiatry: Chromosomes to Community Care.* Wrightson Biomedical Publishing, Petersfield, UK, 1997, pp 143–160.

McGrath AM, Jackson GA. Survey of neuroleptic prescribing in residents of nursing homes in Glasgow. *Br Med J* 1996; 312:611–612.

Schneider LS, Pollock VE, Lyness SA. A meta-analysis of controlled trials of neuroleptic treatment of dementia. *J Am Geriatr Soc* 1990; 38:553–563.

Schneider LS, Sobin PB. Non-neuroleptic medications in the management of agitation in dementia: a selective review. In: E Murphy, G Alexopoulas (eds). *Geriatric Psychiatry: Key Research Topics for Clinicians.* Chichester Publications, London, 1995, pp 127–152.

Spar JE, La Rue A. *Concise Guide to Geriatric Psychiatry,* 2nd edn. American Psychiatric Press, Washington DC, 1997.

Tran-Johnson TK, Krull AJ, Jeste DV. Late life schizophrenia and its treatment: pharmacologic issues in older schizophrenic patients. *Clin Geriatr Med* 1992; 8:401–410.

Wheatley D, Smith D (eds). *Psychopharmacology of Cognitive and Psychiatric Disorders in the Elderly* (*a British Association for Psychopharmacology monograph*). Chapman & Hall Medical, London, 1998.

Zaleon CR, Guthrie SK. Antipsychotic drug use in older adults. *Am J Hosp Pharm* 1994; 51:2917–2943.

Chapter 6

Endocrine Disorders

6.1 DIABETES MELLITUS

6.1.1 Definition and Incidence

Diabetes mellitus is a disorder of carbohydrate metabolism due to a relative or absolute deficiency of insulin. Many older diabetic patients do not present with the classic syndrome of polyuria, polydipsia and polyphagia. They may instead complain of numerous atypical and non-specific symptoms including weight loss, fatigue, anorexia, incontinence, altered sleep pattern and cognitive dysfunction as well as signs and symptoms of typical chronic complications. In the United States, it has been estimated that diabetes mellitus occurs in 18% of persons between 65 and 74 years of age and in as many as 40% of people over 80 years of age. Another 23% of elderly people have impaired glucose tolerance (IGT). Nearly half of all persons known to have type 2 or non-insulin-dependent diabetes mellitus (NIDDM) are over 65 years of age. With improved care and survival the number of elderly insulin-dependent (type 1) diabetics is also rising. Therefore when IGT is included, 40% of the population aged over 65 have some degree of impaired glucose homeostasis.

6.1.2 Making the Diagnosis

If a patient has symptoms of hyperglycaemia (polyuria, polydipsia and weight loss) and unequivocal elevation of plasma glucose (>11.1 mmol/l) on a random laboratory sample, the diagnosis of diabetes mellitus is established. If the patient is asymptomatic, a fasting sample should be obtained. If this is <7.8 mmol/l an oral glucose tolerance test (OGTT) should be performed. If it is >7.8 mmol/l on two occasions the diagnosis is established, if >7.8 mmol/l on one occasion, an OGTT should be performed.

6.1.3 Impaired Glucose Tolerance

It seems likely that a pre-diabetic state occurs in the form of IGT for some time before the onset of frank diabetes. This is defined by the World Health Organization as a fasting venous sample of less than 7.8 mmol/l and a 2 hour postprandial sample of 7.8 to 11.1 after a standardized OGTT with 75 g of glucose. Patients with IGT have twice the normal mortality from strokes, heart attacks and peripheral vascular disease. Unknowingly, patients may continue with IGT for several years and this may explain why many newly diagnosed diabetics have established complications at presentation. The pathogenesis of IGT is complex but may be due in part to a reduced suppression of hepatic glucose. Several factors may be involved in the patient's conversion to frank diabetes including old age, physical inactivity, obesity, higher levels of fasting blood glucose and insulin resistance. Many drugs may also adversely affect glucose tolerance including thiazides, frusemide, beta-blockers, corticosteroids and thyroxine. In a survey of the 10 most widely prescribed drugs in patients aged 75 and over, the most commonly used drug was hydrochlorothiazide. It is important therefore to review the need for such medication in elderly patients with IGT because it may be reversible on cessation of treatment. At present, trials are in progress to determine whether treatment of IGT with oral hypoglycaemics will delay or prevent the onset of frank diabetes and reduce the incidence of macrovascular complications.

6.1.4 Treatment of NIDDM

The therapeutic goals in diabetic patients are to achieve an acceptable blood glucose level, prevent symptoms of uncontrolled hyperglycaemia, avoid hypoglycaemia and prevent or delay the progression of chronic complications of diabetes.

Diet

Diet is the first-line treatment for NIDDM and should be tried on its own for 2 to 3 months unless the patient is highly symptomatic or the response is poor. The advice has been simplified in recent years. Although the ideal diet may be at least 50% of caloric intake from high fibre carbohydrate with fat contributing not more than 35% of energy intake, this may be unrealistic in elderly patients. Simple advice about avoiding cakes, sweets, biscuits and increasing unrefined carbohydrate may be more appropriate.

Oral Hypoglycaemics

Sulphonylureas increase the release of insulin in response to stimulation by glucose. They also upregulate insulin receptors on target tissues, making insulin more effective. They remain first-line agents for the treatment of NIDDM in elderly people and are usually efficacious, at least initially. If low doses do not work it is unlikely that higher doses will be effective. Agents with short half-lives such as **glipizide** (2.5–5 mg daily) and **gliclazide** (40–80 mg daily) should be used in older people because agents with longer half-lives such as chlorpropamide may accumulate and cause severe hypoglycaemia. Glibenclamide may cause similar problems due to selective concentration in islet cells. Therefore **long-acting sulphonylureas should be avoided in elderly patients**. Side-effects such as rashes and blood dyscrasias are uncommon.

Biguanides such as **metformin** reduce hepatic gluconeogenesis and may limit glucose absorption and increase its peripheral uptake. They are useful in obese patients because they suppress appetite. They do not stimulate insulin release and therefore do not cause hypoglycaemia. Their use is limited by a high incidence of gastrointestinal upset, e.g. anorexia, nausea, vomiting, diarrhoea. Lactic acidosis may occasionally occur in association with significant hepatic, renal and cardiac impairment. For this reason metformin should not be used routinely in elderly patients with evidence of renal, liver, cardiac or respiratory impairment. If it is to be used, renal and hepatic function must be checked first and a starting dose of 500 mg daily used initially to minimize side-effects.

Although treatment with sulphonylureas and biguanides will decrease fasting blood glucose levels, postprandial hyperglycaemia persists to a variable degree in about 60% of patients. **Acarbose** competes with dietary oligosaccharides for the digestive alpha-glucosidases in the small intestinal brush border. Binding is reversible so that digestion and absorption of glucose after a meal is slower than normal. Consequently blood glucose concentrations are more stable during the day. Very little acarbose is absorbed and the main side-effects are abdominal distension, flatulence and diarrhoea due to fermentation of unabsorbed carbohydrate in the bowel. This limits its use in many elderly people who cannot tolerate it and may become housebound as a result of the gastrointestinal adverse effects.

Insulin

The natural progression of NIDDM is gradual beta-cell failure. It is estimated that approximately 50% of patients with NIDDM will eventually need insulin. Patients are usually changed to insulin because of poor control on diet and oral hypoglycaemic agents, with or without symptoms of hyperglycaemia. Elderly people in particular may not experience symptoms of thirst, polyuria and weight loss but on closer questioning may admit to tiredness, depression and difficulty with coping with daily tasks, a syndrome known as hyperglycaemic malaise. This may improve significantly with improved glycaemic control with insulin. For this reason insulin should be considered in elderly people in whom fasting blood glucose remains above 9 mmol/l despite optimal diet and oral hypoglycaemic therapy.

Insulin doses are determined on an individual basis by gradually increasing the dose but avoiding troublesome hypoglycaemic reactions. The majority of insulins are now human in type and are prepared biosynthetically. Preparations of human insulin should theoretically be less immunogenic but in trials no real advantage has been shown. There are three main types of insulin preparations: short (soluble insulin and insulin lispro), intermediate (isophane insulin or amorphous insulin zinc suspension) and long acting (insulin zinc suspension–crystalline). Soluble insulin has a rapid onset of action after 30 to 60 minutes, a peak action between 2 and 4 hours and a duration of action up to 8 hours. Insulin lispro is an analogue of human insulin with a more rapid onset, shorter time to peak effect and shorter duration of action than soluble human insulin, which means it can be given before a meal. At present there is no indication for replacing soluble human insulin with insulin lispro but it may help patients whose meal times are unpredictable and in those who eat late and are prone to early nocturnal hypoglycaemia. **The best regimen in elderly patients remains twice daily isophane, e.g. insulatard, or a premixed formulation of soluble and isophane insulin, e.g. mixtard (30% soluble, 70% isophane)**. In a recent study of elderly patients twice daily intermediate-acting insulin regimens were associated with a very low frequency of hypoglycaemia and significant improvement in glycaemic control. Once daily regimens should normally be reserved for very frail patients because administration is easier. However, there is a higher incidence of hypoglycaemia and control is generally less predictable.

6.1.5   Setting Realistic Targets of Therapy

There is justifiable concern that tight glucose control may be associated with an increased risk of symptomatic hypoglycaemia in the elderly. A reasonable practice is to maintain the venous plasma glucose between 5.5 and 11.1 mmol/l. Careful education and follow-up of the elderly diabetic patient is essential. Ideally, this is undertaken by a diabetic peripatetic team, but the appropriate setting for various elements of the programme will vary for any particular patient and between different geographical areas. Certain groups of patients need regular follow-up by specialist hospital teams including those patients maintained on insulin and those who have developed complications.

6.1.6   Acute Diabetic Complications

Hypoglycaemia
Hypoglycaemia is a complication of either sulphonylurea therapy or insulin therapy and often correlates with the rapidity of the fall in glucose level rather than the absolute level. Typical symptoms are:

(i)   Adrenergic-mediated such as tremulousness, anxiety, sweating, palpitations and hunger.
(ii) Neuroglycopenia-mediated such as acute confusion, impaired concentration, personality changes, focal neurological deficits, seizures, syncope and coma.

Older patients usually develop neuroglycopenia symptoms and often develop 'hypoglycaemic unawareness' or do not experience adrenergic symptoms which act as a warning in younger patients. Elderly patients who become hypoglycaemic may be at greater risk of myocardial infarction or cerebrovascular accident because of heightened adrenergic activity. The potential threat and risks of hypoglycaemia are therefore greater in elderly than in younger patients.

Hyperosmolar Non-ketotic Coma (HONK)

One-third to two-thirds of all cases of diabetic hyperosmolar coma occur in patients with no preceding history of diabetes. The predilection of the elderly to hyperosmolar coma may be secondary to age-related impaired maintenance of serum osmolality, decreased thirst sensation or decreased cognitive function interfering with fluid intake. The institu-tionalized immobile elderly patient may lack free access to fluids and may be at even greater risk than community-based independent elderly people. Acute infection is the precipitating cause in 30 to 60% of patients, with pneumonia and urinary tract infections being the most common illnesses. Severe emotional or physical stress, drugs such as thiazides, corticosteroids and phenytoin, poor fluid intake, hypokalaemia and renal failure may also precipitate the condition.

Diabetic hyperosmolar coma is characterized by altered consciousness, marked hyperglycaemia (often >50 mmol/l) and dehydration in the absence of ketoacidosis. Focal neurological deficits may also occur and are usually reversible with correction of the hyperosmolar state. Symptoms start insidiously and may be present for several weeks before presentation. Biochemical characteristics are shown in Table 6.1. The main objective in treatment is to correct the hyperosmolar state, which together with dehydration is the main cause of coma and death. The fluid deficit should be corrected initially with isotonic saline if hypovolaemia is present and the serum sodium is <145 mmol/l. If the serum sodium is ≥145 mmol/l, hypotonic saline is preferable because it delivers more free water. Four to 6 litres may be required to correct the hyperosmolar state but caution is needed in the elderly patient with heart failure or renal insufficiency to avoid fluid overload. Frequent assessment, bladder catheterization and monitoring of central venous pressure is needed. Serum electrolytes should be monitored and hypokalaemia corrected.

Table 6.1   Biochemical characteristics of hyperosmolar coma

Blood glucose 45–60 mmol/l
pH >7.3
Serum bicarbonate >20 mEq/l
Serum osmolality 330–350 mOsm/kg
Anion gap >15 unless lactic acidosis present

Insulin therapy should be started with a low-dose infusion of 0.5 to 1 unit per hour to achieve a reduction of blood glucose of about 10% per hour. When the blood glucose returns to normal, insulin can be given subcutaneously and eventually most patients will maintain glycaemic control with diet or sulphonylurea therapy. However, the condition is often complicated by cerebrovascular accidents, myocardial infarction and venous thromboses which themselves determine the ultimate outcome. Therefore, prophylactic heparin is indicated.

6.1.7   Chronic Diabetic Complications

Vascular complications account for the majority of the morbidity and mortality in diabetic patients. The complications can be divided into three major categories: macrovascular (large vessel disease), microvascular (microangiopathy) and neuropathy. Large vessel disease includes coronary artery disease, stroke and peripheral vascular disease. Coronary and cerebrovascular disease are two to three times more common in diabetics than in the general population. The normal gender protection is lost in elderly females and cardiovascular risk is particularly increased in nephropathy.

Neuropathy
Peripheral nerve damage is common in elderly diabetics. It takes three forms:

(1)   **Autonomic neuropathy** may cause postural hypotension. Precipitants such as tranquillizers, antidepressants and diuretics should be avoided. Graded elastic stockings and fludrocortisone

50–250 mg/day may help. It may also cause gastroparesis characterized by postprandial bloating, nausea, abdominal discomfort and early satiety. Gustatory sweating may also be troublesome. Symptoms can be ameliorated with preprandial metoclopramide or cisapride therapy.

(2) **Sensory neuropathy** is the commonest type and predisposes to diabetic foot ulceration (see below).

(3) **Reversible mononeuropathies and radiculopathies** include proximal femoral neuropathy, cranial nerve palsies and acute painful neuropathies. The condition tends to be self-limiting although symptoms may persist for months or even years. Improving diabetic control is important and even patients with apparently well-controlled NIDDM may need to commence twice daily insulin. Management is otherwise symptomatic. Carbamazepine is sometimes useful for neuropathic pain, and tricyclic antidepressants for insomnia, depression and pain relief.

The Eye

Elderly patients with diabetes may develop deteriorating vision due to cataract, diabetic retinopathy, macular degeneration, glaucoma or retinal vein thrombosis. Up to 20% of newly diagnosed patients with NIDDM have established retinopathy and the proportion affected at diagnosis increases with age. Prevalence of retinopathy increases with duration of diabetes and it primarily affects the macula. Elderly patients with NIDDM should be referred to an ophthalmologist if there is a decline in visual acuity from any cause, fundoscopic evidence of preproliferative, or proliferative retinopathy (with or without vitreous haemorrhage) or lesions indicating early maculopathy, especially the appearance of exudates near the macula. Laser photocoagulation of new vessels in the perimacular area may prevent severe loss of vision.

Diabetes and the Kidney

Diabetic nephropathy affects about 25% of all people with diabetes and is the commonest reason for renal dialysis in the UK and USA. The most important associated risk factor is hypertension, which accelerates progression of diabetic renal disease. Proteinuria is the first sign of diabetic nephropathy and precedes the progressive decline in creatinine clearance that culminates in end-stage renal failure. Diabetic nephropathy with proteinuria is associated with a substantially increased risk of atherosclerosis, which is the main cause of death in older patients.

Routine urinalysis will only detect proteinuria at a concentration of $>300\,\mu g/ml$. However, the threshold for abnormal urinary protein excretion is closer to $20\,\mu g/ml$. Commercial microalbuminuria assays can readily detect clinically significant albuminuria ($>100\,\mu g/ml$) long before urine dipstick tests detect proteinuria and should be used to monitor diabetic patients. There are two main stages in the development of diabetic nephropathy: stage 1 (early or incipient) is associated with raised renal blood flow, raised glomerular filtration rate (GFR) and microalbuminuria. Stage 2 (late or overt) is associated with macroproteinuria, low GFR and raised serum creatinine. Incipient nephropathy is 80% predictive of later development of overt nephropathy and may be reversible. However, once patients have persistent macroproteinuria, progression to renal failure is inevitable. Control of hypertension with angiotensin-converting enzyme (ACE) inhibitors diminishes the rate of protein excretion and slows the decline in renal function in those with overt nephropathy. At the stage of incipient nephropathy, reduction of blood pressure is associated with a reduction in albumin excretion rate and renal protection. However, ACE inhibitors may precipitate acute renal failure in patients with renal artery stenosis, so careful monitoring of renal function, with an initial urea and electrolytes measured after 7–10 days, is essential in the first few months of treatment. Elderly patients with NIDDM in particular need careful assessment before starting treatment with ACE inhibitors. This includes checking for peripheral vascular disease, coronary artery disease or cerebrovascular disease and looking for a disparity in renal size on ultrasound.

Hypertension

Regular measurement of blood pressure is essential in the elderly diabetic patient. Not only will a reduction in blood pressure slow the progression of renal disease but it will also reduce the risks of stroke and heart failure. Blood pressure levels greater than 160/90 in elderly patients need to be treated (see Chapter 2). General measures include reduction in salt and alcohol intake and weight loss. The treatment of choice in diabetics lies between an ACE inhibitor (see above) and a calcium channel antagonist. Alpha-blockers such as doxazosin are also useful, but may be less well tolerated in elderly than in younger patients. Loop diuretics such as frusemide and bumetanide may also be needed in resistant cases. Beta-blockers and thiazide diuretics are relatively contra-indicated in diabetics of all ages.

Diabetic Foot Ulceration

Foot infections/ulceration remain one of the commonest reasons for hospital admissions among diabetic patients. Diabetic foot ulcers result from sensorimotor and autonomic neuropathy, peripheral vascular disease and limited joint mobility. The mainstay of treatment is (1) elevation of the limb to promote venous and lymphatic drainage, (2) diabetic control (usually with twice daily insulin regimens), (3) intra-venous antibiotics for 5 to 7 days followed by a further 14–21 days or longer on oral broad-spectrum antibiotics such as coamoxiclav; metronidazole may be added if the infected ulcer is foul smelling, and (4) occlusive dressings (see Chapter 13). Suitable drug combinations for initial blind therapy of deep tissue infection are amoxycillin plus flucloxacillin and metronidazole or ciprofloxacin and metronidazole. Clindamycin is suitable where there is suspected or definite osteo-myelitis, but carries a considerable risk of pseudomembranous colitis. Patients need to be educated about foot care, regular chiropathy and appropriate dressings. They should be advised to bathe their feet daily, drying well between the toes. They should avoid hot water bottles, see a chiropodist regularly and use appropriate footwear. An effective way to provide care for high-risk individuals is at a combined foot clinic where patients will see a physician, vascular surgeon, shoe fitter, chiropodist and nurse.

6.1.8   Prevention of Diabetic Complications

Large Vessel Disease

In diabetic patients several cardiac risk factors often coexist, e.g. glucose intolerance, hypertension and an abnormal lipid profile, which may act synergistically to increase cardiovascular risk. Insulin resistance may underlie all of these conditions. In addition, diabetic patients may smoke. The principles for prevention and treatment are the same as for the non-diabetic population (see Chapter 2).

Microangiopathy

Strict glycaemic control at an early age in young-onset IDDM patients delays the onset and slows the progression of retinopathy, neuropathy and nephropathy, although at the increased risk of hypoglycaemia. Unfortunately, the effect of tight diabetic control on progression of complications in elderly NIDDM patients is not known, nor is there any evidence of advantages from the use of insulin rather than oral hypoglycaemic agents.

6.2 THYROID DISEASE IN THE ELDERLY

Thyroid disease, especially hypothyroidism, is one of the most common endocrine conditions of elderly people. However, the atypical presentation of both hypo- and hyperthyroidism in this age group may mean the diagnosis is not considered. On the other hand, evidence from community studies suggests that general screening of the population for thyroid disease detects few cases and is therefore unjustified, even in high-risk groups such as women over 60. Thyroid function should not therefore be assessed in entirely fit and active elderly people.

Thyroid function tests (TFTs) may be difficult to interpret in patients with non-thyroidal illness, particularly if they are taking concomitant drug treatment, and a diagnosis should not be made until the TFTs are repeated 6 weeks after resolution of an acute illness. In acutely ill patients the plasma TSH level is reduced, particularly in those with a low energy intake or those receiving treatment with corticosteroids or dopamine, but it often rises during convalescence and may be transiently raised above the normal range. Total serum thyroxine (T4) may be low due to reduced synthesis and impaired binding to plasma proteins by free fatty acids. Although this causes an increase in free T4, hyperthyroidism does not occur because of reduced cellular uptake in T4 and reduced conversion to tri-iodothyronine (T3). Several drugs may also cause abnormal thyroid function tests, e.g. propranolol, amiodarone, oestrogen (increased total T4) and phenytoin, diclogenac and corticosteroids (reduced total T4).

Despite these difficulties, the threshold for screening elderly patients for thyroid disease should be low because it is common in this age group. If patients are very ill, however, TFTs should not be done unless there is clinical suspicion of thyroid disease and a concern that hyper- or hypothyroidism may be definitely contributing to the clinical condition. In elderly patients with vague or non-specific symptoms in the absence of overt acute illness, thyroid testing is required to detect clinically unrecognized thyroid dysfunction. The most reliable test in the absence of non-thyroidal illness is the serum thyroid-stimulating hormone (TSH) concentration.

6.2.1 Hypothyroidism

Primary failure of the thyroid gland is responsible for the vast majority of elderly hypothyroid cases. It usually develops insidiously after years of undiagnosed chronic autoimmune thyroiditis. Hypothyroidism can also result from iatrogenic causes such as previous treatment of hyperthyroidism with radioactive iodine, ingestion of antithyroid drugs such as iodides and lithium and, occasionally, thyroid surgery. Less than a third of older adults show typical signs and symptoms such as cold intolerance and weight gain. Instead, they may present with non-specific symptoms of malaise, fatigue, failing health, falling, incontinence, psychomotor retardation, cognitive impairment, psychosis and depression. Myxoedema coma may occasionally be caused by non-compliance with thyroxine or use of respiratory depressants such as opiates and phenothiazines. Hypothyroidism is diagnosed in the presence of a raised TSH and a low free T4. If the T4 is normal and the patient has a history of goitre, previous treatment with radioactive iodine or is on lithium or amiodarone, replacement with L-thyroxine should be considered if the TSH is >10 mU/l. If the patient has none of these predisposing features, the test should be repeated in 4 to 6 weeks and treatment started then if the TSH level is >10 mU/l. If TSH is <10 mU/l, thyroid peroxidase (microsomal) antibodies should be measured to help distinguish those with underlying thyroid disease. Those patients with positive antibodies should be treated with thyroxine because the conversion rate from subclinical to overt hypothyroidism is at least 5% per year.

The starting dose of thyroxine in elderly patients is 25 µg daily to avoid worsening ischaemic heart disease or arrhythmias. Gradual dosage increments of 25 µg daily can be made at 4 to 6 week intervals, with serum T4 and TSH measured at the end of each interval. Although the therapeutic end point is normalization of T4 and TSH concentrations, this may not be possible in those patients in whom higher doses cause a deterioration in cardiovascular symptoms. The usual maintenance dose in the elderly is 50 to 100 µg per day. It is important to avoid iatrogenic hyperthyroidism (i.e. subnormal TSH levels) because of the risk of precipitating arrhythmias, cardiac failure and weight loss.

6.2.2   Hyperthyroidism

Hyperthyroidism in old age can be subtle and, like hypothyroidism, often lacks the specific presenting signs seen in younger patients. In elderly patients the commonest features are tachycardia, fatigue and weight loss. Atrial fibrillation is the presenting disorder in one-third of cases. Ten to 15% of patients with thyrotoxicosis are over 60 years. The syndrome of 'apathetic thyrotoxicosis' is almost exclusively a disease of elderly people. The patient presents with weakness, lethargy, depression and muscle wasting and lacks the typical features of hyperactivity, irritability, sweating and tremulousness.

A suppressed serum TSH concentration is indicative of hyperthyroidism except when the patient is on dopamine, high dose corticosteroids or somatostatin or has intercurrent non-thyroidal illness. The finding of a low TSH should be followed by measurement of free T4, which will be raised in thyrotoxicosis but may also be raised in non-thyroidal disease. In this situation a raised serum T3 is indicative of thyrotoxicosis.

Graves' disease is an uncommon form of thyrotoxicosis in elderly people who often lack the classic exophthalmic, skin, goitre or hyperadrenergic features. The principal cause of hyperthyroidism in this age group is a single toxic adenoma or a toxic multinodular goitre. Iodine-induced hyperthyroidism may occur in non-toxic multinodular goitre when patients are exposed to radiocontrast material containing iodine, cough syrups or amiodarone. De Quervain's thyroiditis is characterized by a moderately enlarged thyroid gland, raised erythrocyte sedimentation rate and transient thyrotoxicosis. Finally, a common cause of hyperthyroidism in old age is inappropriate or excessive treatment with thyroxine.

Antithyroid Drugs

The thiourea derivatives (carbimazole and propylthiouracil) are no longer recommended as sole therapy for Graves' disease in elderly adults. Radioiodine is the mainstay of treatment in cases of toxic adenoma and Graves' disease but antithyroid drugs are given to achieve euthyroidism first. Once daily treatment with carbimazole makes it the drug of choice. A typical starting dose is 15 to 20 mg daily. It is then titrated down against serum thyroxine concentrations checked at 4 to 6 week intervals until a maintenance dose of 5 to 15 mg daily is achieved to keep T4 in the normal range. TSH measurement is unhelpful during the first 3 months of treatment but thereafter a sudden rise above normal may indicate iatrogenic hypothyroidism. The most serious, although uncommon, adverse effect of carbimazole treatment is agranulocytosis, which is more common in the elderly. It may have a rapid onset, making routine leucocyte counts unreliable screening tools. Patients should be advised to report immediately if they develop fever, sore throat or malaise. Therapy should be stopped, the patient hospitalized and infection treated aggressively if neutropenia is identified. Agranulocytosis and other rare side-effects such as hepatitis and lupus-like syndromes represent absolute contraindications to carbimazole. Rashes are common but often resolve on continuing treatment. If rashes continue, propylthiouracil may be substituted but can also cause agranulocytosis.

Beta-blockers may be used as adjunctive treatment to control hyperthyroid-induced hypertension, tachycardia, palpitation or tremor but are contraindicated in the presence of asthma, heart failure or peripheral vascular disease.

Radioiodine

For most elderly patients with persisting thyrotoxicosis a single 5–10 mCi dose of radioactive iodine is the treatment of choice, repeated after 6 months if necessary. Carbimazole is discontinued for several days before radioiodine and resumed several days after treatment. It is continued until the patient is euthyroid following the radioiodine and then gradually withdrawn. The incidence of hypothyroidism is 2 to 3% per year following radioiodine. Radioiodine must be used with caution in patients with Graves' disease with ophthalmopathy because there is a significant risk of exacerbation of eye problems. Toxic adenomata and toxic multinodular goitres are treated with radioiodine preceded by antithyroid drugs. Predominant nodules in a multinodular gland should be evaluated for malignancy with fine needle biopsy.

Surgery
Surgery is reserved as definitive therapy for Graves' disease for occasional patients who decline radioiodine or suffer local compressive symptoms in the neck or superior mediastinum.

Thyrotoxic Crisis
This is a life-threatening medical emergency in the thyrotoxic elderly patient precipitated by infection, trauma or other physiological stress. It is characterized by fever, hypertension, tachycardia and agitation, and is associated with a 20% mortality rate. Treatment is with high doses of propylthiouracil (150–300 mg) followed by intravenous sodium iodide (1–2 g/24 h after at least 1 hour) and beta-blockers. Anticoagulation may be indicated if the patient is in atrial fibrillation.

6.3 OESTROGEN HORMONE REPLACEMENT THERAPY (HRT) IN OLD AGE

In postmenopausal women oestrogen replacement therapy is recommended for prevention and treatment of osteoporosis and is thought to reduce the incidence of coronary and cerebrovascular disease. Oestrogen replacement therapy can improve the elasticity, moisture and thickness of vaginal, perineal and periurethral tissues, improving symptoms of vaginal dryness, dyspareunia and urinary urgency. Unless the uterus has been removed surgically, HRT should include a progestogen compound to minimize the risk of endometrial hyperplasia and carcinoma. HRT is contraindicated in patients with unexplained vaginal bleeding, recent history of deep venous thrombosis, pulmonary embolus, breast or endometrial carcinoma or a family history of an oestrogen-dependent neoplasm.

To derive maximum benefit in terms of osteoporosis prevention HRT should be introduced as early after menopause as possible. Questions have been posed about the rationale for initiating HRT in women who are many years post menopause. However, elderly women who present with evidence of osteoporosis should still be considered for HRT. Likewise, therapy should be considered in women at risk from cardio-vascular disease, or who have had early surgical menopause. It is uncertain whether women who have started HRT in the early postmeno-pausal period should continue it indefinitely. However, the evidence suggests that although the greatest reduction in hip fracture rates occur in women who begin HRT soon after menopause, women older than 70 still continue to benefit. Therefore continuing HRT indefinitely may be appropriate, particularly in women who already have osteoporosis.

Retrospective studies suggest that women taking unopposed oestrogens have a reduced incidence of coronary heart disease which is possibly related to oestrogen-related changes in lipoprotein profile, glucose metabolism or blood pressure. The effect of the added progestogen on cardiovascular risk is unknown but at least some of those used in HRT decrease high density lipoprotein (HDL) and increase low density lipoprotein (LDL). In women at high risk of coronary artery disease, there is a case for treatment with unopposed oestrogens, even when the uterus is intact, provided that endometrial biopsies are performed at yearly intervals. Alternatively, a progestogen such as medroxyprogester-one, which does not adversely affect lipids, may be used to produce menstruation, which is usually light.

6.3.1 HRT Regimens

The primary components of most HRT preparations are one or more natural oestrogens. These include oestradiol, oestrone, oestriol and conjugated equine oestrogens. The progestogens used are synthetically produced and differ structurally from naturally occurring progesterone and include dydrogesterone, medroxyprogesterone acetate, levonorges-trel, norgestrel and norethisterone. The commonest regimens for post-menopausal women with intact uteri are continuous-combined and cyclic-combined oestrogen and progestogen, usually in tablet form. Continuous-combined HRT is associated with less breakthrough bleed-ing but patients may be troubled more by side-effects (see below) from the progestogen. During 28-day cyclical treatment, progestogens are given for 10–14 days, so producing monthly withdrawal bleeding. During 3-monthly cyclical treatment progestogens are given for 14 days with the aim of producing quarterly withdrawal bleed. Such cyclical treatment minimizes the development of oestrogen-induced endometrial hyperplasia.

Another option is transdermal administration of oestradiol, which may have advantages in that it reduces first-pass metabolism and has no known effects on thrombosis. It may be better tolerated in patients with nausea or occasional migraine headaches. It is associated with mild skin irritation in 25 to 30% of patients with blistering in a small proportion of patients. Two types of transdermal patch are currently available. The earlier version releases the oestrogen from an in-built reservoir and has an adhesive outer ring. In the newer type the oestrogen is evenly distributed throughout the adherent part of the patch. Oestradiol can also be applied to the skin in the form of a gel dispensed from a pressurized container. Crystalline pellets of oestradiol (implants) can be inserted subcutaneously under local anaesthetic providing continuous oestrogen therapy for several months. An oral progestogen must be taken if the woman still has her uterus.

Adverse Effects

Oestrogen-related side-effects include nausea, breast tenderness and headaches. The nausea is often self-limiting and resolves within the first 2 months of therapy. The effect may be diminished by taking the medication with food or at bedtime. Some patients will benefit from switching to another oestrogen preparation or using transdermal oestrogen instead of tablets. Rarely a patient cannot tolerate the ideal dosage level and a lower dose of oestrogen may be used initially. This may also alleviate breast tenderness. Other solutions to breast tenderness are to omit HRT for a few days at the end of each month, thereby giving the patient an oestrogen break, to reduce caffeine and to switch to another progestogen. Migraine is a relative contraindication to HRT. New headaches in a patient on HRT should be investigated fully. There is also a very small but significantly increased risk of breast cancer from use of HRT (relative risk 1.023 whilst taking HRT or within 4 years of stopping therapy, according to one recent large-scale meta-analysis). After 5 years of cessation of use, there is no increased risk.

Adverse effects due to the progestogen include mood swings, abdominal bloating and constipation. Mood swings may be alleviated by prescribing a different progestogen or a lower dose of drug. Abdominal bloating may respond to a change in progestogen preparation.

Postmenopausal Bleeding

Continuous-combined treatment induces amenorrhoea in over 75% of women within 6 months. Irregular uterine bleeding may occur during the first 4–6 months of treatment with continuous regimens. Such symptoms usually do not warrant investigation unless uterine bleeding is getting heavier rather than lighter, persists for more than 6 months or continues after stopping the treatment. Any bleeding that occurs after prolonged amenorrhoea should be investigated by endometrial curettage. Bleeding that occurs at the time of progestogen withdrawal in a cyclic-combined regimen is usually due to hormonal stimulation of the endometrium. Bleeding that occurs irregularly throughout the treatment cycle should be evaluated by endometrial biopsy. Patients with other risk factors for endometrial carcinoma (obesity, hypertension, diabetes, nulliparity, early menarche or late menopause) should have endometrial biopsy regardless of the timing of the bleeding. If there is no evidence of atypical endometrial cells the dose of progestogen may be increased and the biopsy repeated after 6 months. If there is any evidence of cellular atypia, dilatation and curettage is indicated to look for endometrial carcinoma.

Alternative Agents

Tibolone, a synthetic oral steroid with oestrogenic, progestogenic and androgenic actions, is a licensed alternative to oestrogen HRT which can control menopausal symptoms. It can prevent bone mineral loss but is not licensed for the prevention of osteoporosis and it is not known whether it reduces the risk of coronary artery disease. It is contra-indicated in women with hormone-dependent malignancy.

6.4 HYPERCALCAEMIA

A wide range of diseases can cause hypercalcaemia but in clinical practice about 90% of cases are caused by primary hyperparathyroidism or malignancy (Table 6.2). In the primary care setting, primary hyper-

Table 6.2   Causes of hypercalcaemia

Primary hyperparathyroidism	
Malignant disease	Humoral hypercalcaemia of malignancy Metastatic bone disease Multiple myeloma
Other	Hyperthyroidism Addison's disease Thiazides Vitamin A or D toxicity

Table 6.3   Clinical features of hypercalcaemia

Neuropsychiatric	Lethargy, headache, confusion, sleep disturbance, depression, altered level of consciousness, drowsiness, stupor, coma
Gastrointestinal	Anorexia, nausea, vomiting, constipation, acute pancreatitis
Renal	Polyuria, polydipsia, nocturia, hypercalciuria, nephrocalcinosis
Cardiological	Arrhythmias
Musculoskeletal	Arthralgia, muscle weakness
Eyes	Corneal calcification
Skin	Pruritus

parathyroidism is the most common cause whilst in the hospital environment malignancy is commoner. Many symptoms and signs may be caused by hypercalcaemia (Table 6.3). Total serum calcium must be corrected for low albumin by adding or subtracting 0.02 mmol/l for every 1 g/l albumin below or above an albumin concentration of 40 g/l. Alkaline phosphatase will be increased in patients with hyperparathyroidism (if there is bone involvement) and most forms of malignant hypercalcaemia. It is often normal in myeloma and some forms of lymphoma.

6.4.1   Emergency Treatment for Malignant Hypercalcaemia or Parathyroid Crisis

This is indicated for patients with significant hypercalcaemic symptoms or who have a serum calcium more than 3.5 mmol/l. Any drugs such as thiazides which might be contributing to the hypercalcaemia should be stopped. Treatment should comprise:

(1) *Rehydration.* Severely hypercalcaemic patients are often profoundly dehydrated and intravenous isotonic saline is the most appropriate fluid replacement. Patients may be depleted of 5–10 litres of extracellular fluid and a replacement of 3–4 litres in the first 24 hours is appropriate, with central venous pressure monitoring if necessary. Frusemide is not routinely used unless the patient becomes volume overloaded or has cardiac failure. Special caution is recommended when replacing large volumes of fluid in this age group.

(2) *Bisphosphonates.* These are the drugs of choice to be combined with rehydration. Pamidronate 60 mg given in 3 litres of isotonic saline as a single infusion over 24 hours may be used. An alternative is clodronate. Both drugs should be used with caution in patients with renal impairment but are safe in patients having adequate rehydration.

(3) *Calcitonin and glucocorticoids.* In patients with malignant hypercalcaemia and renal failure, where bisphosphonates and large fluid volumes are relatively contraindicated, calcitonin 200 units every 12 hours subcutaneously combined with 100 mg of hydrocortisone given every 6 hours will reduce serum calcium in most patients.

(4) *Dialysis.* This is occasionally necessary for patients with severe hypercalcaemia who are in renal failure.

FURTHER READING

Bilezikian JP. Management of acute hypercalcaemia. *N Engl J Med* 1992; 326:1196–1203.

Evans MP, Fleming KC, Evans JM. Hormone replacement therapy: Management of common problems. *Mayo Clin Proc: Symposium on Geriatrics* 1995; 70:800–805.

Finucane P, Sinclair AJ. *Diabetes in Old Age.* John Wiley & Sons, Chichester, 1995.

Rae P, Farrar, J, Beckett G, Toft A. Assessment of thyroid status in elderly people. *Br Med J* 1993; 307:177–180.

Singh I, Marshall MC. Diabetes mellitus in the elderly. *Endocrinol Metab Clin North Am* 1995; 24:255–272.

Vanderpump MPJ, Ahlquist JAO, Franklyn JA, Clayton RN. Consensus statement for good practice and audit measures in the management of hypothyroidism and hyperthyroidism. *Br Med J* 1996; 313:539–544.

Chapter 7

Nutritional and Gastrointestinal Disorders

7.1 NUTRITIONAL DISORDERS

The body mass index (BMI) is the best method of describing an adult's nutritional status. It is defined by the weight (kg) divided by the height squared (m^2). Optimal BMI ranges between 20 and 25 kg/m^2. A BMI of $<20 \, kg/m^2$ suggests malnutrition and values less than 18 kg/m^2 confirm malnutrition. Malnutrition has important consequences for people of all ages, such as reduced physical function due to muscle weakness and atrophy, apathy and cognitive impairment, reduced immune function with susceptibility to infections and other physiological stresses, poor wound healing, increased risk of pressure sores and prolonged hospitalization. Overall hospital mortality is significantly increased among malnourished patients compared to those with normal nutritional status.

Protein–calorie malnutrition is a common problem in elderly people. Surveys of community-dwelling elderly people report a steady prevalence rate increase from 3% among all those over 65 to about 15% of those over 80 years. The prevalence of malnutrition is even higher in hospitalized elderly. A recent survey of 500 consecutive people admitted to a UK hospital reported that 40% of these patients had a BMI less than 20 kg/m^2, 14% had a BMI of 16–18 kg/m^2 and 9% had a BMI less than 16 kg/m^2. At discharge follow-up of 112 patients, there was a mean weight loss of 5.4% compared to admission, most marked among those who were most malnourished. Elderly institutionalized people have an even higher likelihood of malnutrition (approximately 50–80%). Like most syndromes in old people, malnutrition is usually multifactorial, with intrinsic and extrinsic aetiological factors contributing to the overall problem. Intrinsic factors include reduced appetite and smell, edentulousness and ill-fitting dentures, physical disability leading to problems with food preparation, immobility, cognitive impairment, depression, ignorance regarding nutrition, multiple illnesses and medications, and malabsorption. Extrinsic factors include reduced income and social isolation: people who eat alone consume less food. Careful documentation of these risk factors is important, since many are remediable.

The daily nutrition requirements of healthy elderly people are: (i) energy 25–30 kcal/kg; (ii) protein 0.8 g/kg; (iii) iron 10 mg; (iv) calcium 1000 mg; (v) vitamin D 800 IU; (vi) vitamin C 60 mg; (vii) folic acid 200 µg. Ageing per se is not associated with significantly reduced absorption of nutrients. Malnourished elderly people and those suffering from trauma and sepsis usually have greater requirements. Sick elderly people usually do not manage to eat full meals but sometimes manage to meet their nutritional requirements with frequent snacks outside mealtimes, particularly if the calorific content of the food intake is maximized, for example by lipid-rich additives like cream or butter. If protein–calorie intake is still inadequate, **nutritional supplements** may be necessary. These should be appetizing, energy-rich liquids or semi-solid feeds with sufficient essential nutrients. Oral supplements result in fewer wound problems in malnourished patients awaiting elective surgery, significant reductions in morbidity and mortality rates in elderly patients with fractured neck of femur when taken during the first month of hospitalization and a 10% reduction in all-cause mortality when taken for up to 6 months in elderly people receiving long-term nursing care.

Table 7.1 summarizes the important aspects of nutritional evaluation in old people. Malnutrition should be corrected vigorously and often requires the input of the multidisciplinary rehabilitation team other than the dietician, e.g. the occupational therapist if there are problems with managing drinking vessels or cutlery, the medical social worker if organization of meals-on-wheels is required, the dentist if dental/oral health problems impinge on patients' ability to eat. There is no good evidence that any one particular type of nutritional supplement is more beneficial than others in elderly people with malnutrition. However, certain types of nutritional supplement will benefit certain patients, e.g. high protein supplements in patients with major sepsis, high lipid and high fibre supplements in diabetic patients with marked hyperglycaemia, and high fibre supplements in those suffering from diarrhoea related to tube feeding (by virtue of increasing bulk in the diet, e.g. ispaghula husk). Successful nutritional supplementation is determined as much by patient preference as by differential nutritional content, so it is important to make sure that the individual formula offered is palatable. As with all malnourished patients starting nutritional replacement, elderly patients may experience electrolyte abnormalities, hyperglycaemia and hypotension which can be minimized by appropriate biochemical and clinical monitoring.

Artificial feeding techniques, such as by nasogastric tube and enterostomy, have associated morbidity (principally aspiration) and should be avoided where possible in elderly people. However, in certain situations (mainly dysphagia or profound anorexia), deteriorating nutritional status coupled with inability to maintain adequate oral intake make tube feeding necessary if further functional decline and death are to be prevented. Early intervention with **nasogastric tube** (NGT) feeding, particularly in elderly malnourished patients with post-stroke dysphagia (and the prospect of functional improvement), fractured neck of femur and those awaiting elective abdominal surgery is beneficial. If enteral feeding is required for more than 4–6 weeks, **percutaneous endoscopic gastrostomy** (PEG) is preferred to NGT feeding, mainly because of

Table 7.1 Nutritional assessment in old people

(1) Body mass index (BMI = weight (kg) ÷ height $(m)^2$)
    BMI <18 → malnutrition; BMI >27 → obesity (optimal BMI 20–25 kg/m^2)

(2) Weight loss >10% of normal body weight in the previous 6 months is significant and requires investigation

(3) Useful laboratory indices of malnutrition
    (i) Serum albumin <35 g/l
    (ii) Serum cholesterol <4.65 mmol/l (180 mg/dl)
    (iii) Total lymphocyte count <1.5×10^9

(4) Malnutrition risk factor assessment
    (i) Low income
    (ii) Living alone/socially isolated
    (iii) Depression/dementia
    (iv) Multiple pathology/poor physical function
    (v) Polypharmacy
    (vi) Poor dentition

better patient tolerability and safety. There is also limited evidence showing improved survival and shorter duration of hospitalization in elderly stroke patients randomized to PEG feeding compared with NGT feeding. **Intravenous parenteral nutrition** is seldom required, is expensive and is associated with septicaemia due to central venous catheter infection. Therefore, it is reserved for malnourished patients whose gastrointestinal absorption is severely impaired as a result of disease or surgery.

Specific syndromes resulting from specific **vitamin and trace element deficiencies** are well-described, and elderly people are at greatest risk. Often, symptoms and signs are subtle, and are wrongly attributed to 'just old age'. Examples include the painful red, smooth mouth and tongue and seborrheic dermatitis associated with riboflavin deficiency, the '3 Ds' of niacin deficiency (photosensitive dermatitis, dementia and deranged bowel habit), and the bruising and poor wound healing associated with vitamin C deficiency (scurvy). Thiamine (vitamin B_1) deficiency is seen occasionally in elderly people, particularly where there is a history of alcohol abuse. Wernicke's encephalopathy (delirium, ataxia and ophthalmoplegia) is particularly likely to occur if glucose is infused intravenously before thiamine is given; therefore, thiamine and glucose should always be given together in alcoholic patients. There is little point in embarking on complex investigations of specific vitamin deficiencies (other than vitamin B_{12}) when the dietary history confirms poor nutritional intake. Broad-spectrum vitamin supplementation for 2–3 weeks will usually and rapidly correct vitamin deficiency symptoms until normal, balanced dietary intake of food is re-established.

Obesity is less of a problem in elderly people than malnutrition. It is defined by a BMI >27%. Severe obesity (>130% of desirable body weight) is associated with immobility, sleep apnoea, diabetes mellitus, osteoarthritis of the hips and knees, thromboembolism, hypertension, pressure sores and intertrigo. Most examples of morbid obesity result from overeating. Occasional cases result from endocrine disorders, glucocorticoids and long-term phenothiazines. Calorie restriction to not less than 800 kcal/day, with adequate supplementation of vitamins and minerals, coupled with gentle aerobic exercise, is appropriate for elderly obese patients. 'Slimming drugs', such as fenfluramine and L-thyroxine (in euthyroid persons), are best avoided.

7.2 ORAL CAVITY DISORDERS

Dental caries, periodontal disease and edentulousness are common problems in old age. **Dental caries** and **periodontal disease** are associated with loosening of teeth and painful, swollen gums that may bleed easily. Established periodontal disease is virtually impossible to eradicate. Chronic gingival inflammation is followed by separation of the gum from the tooth, which eventually leads to tooth loosening. Advanced periodontal disease may be associated with bacteraemia during mastication, with potentially serious consequences for patients with valvular heart disease and internal prostheses of various types, e.g. prosthetic cardiac valves, prosthetic hip joints. Periodontal disease may be held in check by regular dental scaling and the use of plastic fibres impregnated with tetracyclines, supplemented by antiseptic mouthwashes (e.g. chlorhexidine gluconate 0.1% 10–15 ml in a glass of lukewarm water two to three times daily). Severely carious teeth should be extracted, particularly in frail elderly people, in whom there is a risk of dental fracture or dislodgement with aspiration, or where sharp teeth are interfering with food intake. **Halitosis** may also be treated effectively with dilute chlorhexidine mouthwash two to three times daily.

Dentures may be associated with traumatic mouth ulcers, slipping (resulting in poor mastication of food) and a variety of less common long-term problems, such as epulis, leucoplakia and squamous carcinoma. Dentures may also act as a reservoir for infecting microorganisms, such as *Candida albicans*. Dentures should always be removed at night-time, cleaned and disinfected. Sodium hypochlorite 10% solution (dilute household bleach or Milton fluid) is a suitable denture disinfectant.

Xerostomia, or salivary insufficiency, may result in problems with chewing, speaking and dental caries, as well as cause an uncomfortable burning sensation in the mouth. It is usually a side-effect of drugs with anticholinergic properties, such as tricyclic antidepressants (see Chapter 5) and drugs for bladder detrusor instability (see Chapter 10). Sometimes, it results from Sjögren's syndrome or damage to salivary glands from surgery or irradiation. Xerostomia may be successfully relieved by use of artificial saliva products (e.g. Luborant 2–3 sprays up to four times daily). Sugarless lemon drops and chewing gums may also help.

Acutely painful mouth ulcers commonly result from candidal infections and aphthae. **Oral candidiasis** is associated with antibiotic therapy, immunodeficiency, corticosteroid therapy, diabetes mellitus, xerostomia and ill-fitting dentures. Candidal infection may present as soft, white plaques which reveal underlying bleeding points when removed, or as numerous, extremely painful white lesions with a red halo. Where diagnosis is uncertain, oral swabbing for microbiological confirmation may be helpful. **Nystatin suspension** (100 000 units/ml) or **pastilles**, **clotrimazole gel**, **amphotericin lozenges or suspension** are all effective in oral candidiasis. Nystatin suspension should be rinsed around the mouth for several minutes four to six times daily and swallowed. Therapy should be continued for 14 days. Dentures should be carefully disinfected in cases of confirmed oral candidiasis to avoid relapse. **Angular cheilitis** may result from ill-fitting dentures or vitamin B complex deficiency. More recent evidence indicates that chronic, low-grade candidal infection is often important. Local topical anticandidal therapy (e.g. combined miconazole 2% and hydrocortisone 1%; Daktacort) may be very helpful in clearing this often painful lesion, with eradication of intraoral candidiasis where it coexists. Sometimes, there is associated *Staphylococcus aureus* infection in the lesions, in which case externally applied clioquinol-hydrocortisone cream (Vioform HC) may be beneficial.

Aphthous ulcers are typically recurrent, appear white in the base with an erythematous margin, are smooth and are usually found on oral mucosa remote from the periosteum. They are disproportionately painful to their size. They usually heal spontaneously in 5–10 days. Frequent, recurrent attacks should raise the possibility of underlying, immunologically mediated disorders, such as inflammatory bowel disease, coeliac disease and Behçet's syndrome. The diagnosis is usually clearcut when attacks are recurrent, but the possibility of herpetic ulceration should be considered with isolated attacks of multifocal oral ulceration. Aphthous ulcers respond well to **hydrocortisone lozenges** (2.5 mg four times daily; Corlan). In severe cases, **triamcinolone acetonide** 0.1% oral paste (Adcortyl in Orabase) applied gently over the lesions two to four times daily may be tried; it should not be used for more than 5 days to avoid adrenocortical suppression and other corticosteroid side-effects.

Herpes labialis is not uncommonly associated with serious infections in elderly people, particularly pneumococcal pneumonia. The diagnosis is usually made when the lesions become clinically obvious, by which time acyclovir topically or by tablet does not reduce the symptoms or duration of the ulcers any more than placebo. Simple analgesics and topical antibiotic ointments for secondary impetiginization, if it occurs, are appropriate.

7.3 SWALLOWING AND OESOPHAGEAL DISORDERS

The term 'presbyoesophagus' has been used to refer to the principal functional changes in the elderly oesophagus, and encompasses reduced amplitude of peristaltic contractions, frequent tertiary contractions, delayed oesophageal emptying, incomplete sphincter relaxation and oesophageal dilatation. However, it is not clear whether these changes are attributable to age-related comorbid diseases or the ageing process itself. Ageing is associated an increased incidence of **dysphagia**, of both the transfer and transport types. **Transfer dysphagia** refers to problems with transfer of food or liquid from the mouth to the proximal oesophagus and commonly results from neuromuscular disorders, mainly cerebrovascular disease, Parkinson's disease, thyroid dysfunction, motor neurone disease and systemic myopathies. **Transport dysphagia** usually indicates oesophageal obstruction, due to peptic stricture or carcinoma most commonly. Occasionally, transport dysphagia results from disorders of peristaltic function (e.g. achalasia of the cardia, oesophageal spasm), Zenker's diverticulum, paraoesophageal hernia, extrinsic neck or mediastinal tumours, Schatski's ring (invaginated gastro-oesophageal mucosa) and extrinsic aortic aneurysmal compression. Oesophageal stricture may sometimes be drug-induced, from ulceration due to non-steroidal anti-inflammatory drugs (NSAIDs), potassium chloride tablets and tetracycline.

The management of each of these causes of transport dysphagia is beyond the scope of this book, but is generally no different in elderly than in younger patients. Many elderly people understate chronic dysphagic symptoms and wrongly attribute them to longstanding indigestion or 'just old age'. Elderly patients respond equally well to oesophageal dilatation as young people and seldom require definitive corrective surgery (as younger patients may do). Patients of all ages should be followed up carefully, since elderly patients are at greater risk of fatal aspiration and repeat dilatation is often required at intervals of 6–12 months. Palliation of **malignant, inoperable oesophageal strictures** is effective in elderly as well as young patients. Dysphagia and malnutrition from malignant oesophageal stricture may respond very well to endoscopic dilatation or laser therapy or placement of prosthetic tubes (e.g. Atkinson tube). Oesophageal cancer has a very poor prognosis, despite attempts at cure with surgery, radiotherapy and chemotherapy, with an overall 5-year survival rate of 5–10%.

Gastro-oesophageal reflux (GOR) is a common problem in elderly people, although it is not always symptomatic. The increased prevalence of GOR in old age is attributable to presbyoesophagus, increased prevalence of hiatus hernia and conditions that cause raised intra-abdominal pressure (e.g. obesity, respiratory illness leading to chronic cough, chronic prostatism). Certain drugs may impair lower oesophageal sphincter closing function, such as nitrates, calcium channel blockers, anticholinergics, nicotine, alcohol and caffeine. Typical symptoms of posture-related heartburn with rapid relief from antacids may be absent in old people, who may present with late complications of longstanding GOR, such as stricture. In symptomatic patients, first-line therapy is with **antacids** or **alginates** (e.g. Gaviscon liquid 10 ml 30–60 minutes after meals plus nocte), which are effective in most patients.

Breakthrough GOR symptoms may be treated with additional **H$_2$-antagonists**, best given at bedtime. Cimetidine 800 mg nocte is generally suitable, and is as effective as the other H$_2$-antagonists for both healing of oesophagitis and control of reflux symptoms. However, cimetidine inhibits the hepatic cytochrome P450 enzyme system so that caution is required when prescribing it with other drugs that are metabolized by this enzyme system (e.g. warfarin, theophylline, phenytoin). Potential adverse drug interactions may be less of a problem with the other H$_2$-antagonists, such as ranitidine. Persistent symptoms may be helped by addition of prokinetic agents, such as **metoclopramide** 10 mg three times daily. Domperidone 10 mg four times daily or cisapride 10 mg four times daily are alternatives, but are no more effective than metoclopramide and are substantially more expensive. The most effective therapy for relapsed, refractory symptomatic GOR is a **proton pump inhibitor** (e.g. omeprazole 20–40 mg nocte, lansoprazole 30–60 mg nocte). They are very well tolerated drugs and seldom cause significant problems with adverse drug interactions. However, they are expensive and the marked hypo-/achlorhydria from their use may impair iron and vitamin B_{12} absorption, which can lead to overt deficiency in patients with borderline haematinic stores. It is often possible to abolish GOR symptoms and endoscopic oesphagitis with maintenance low doses of omeprazole (10 mg nocte) or lansoprazole (15 mg nocte). Surgery is seldom indicated or successful for severe GOR.

Chronic GOR is associated with increased risk of **Barrett's epithelium**, i.e. columnar metaplasia of the distal oesophagus. Patients with Barrett's epithelium have an increased risk of malignancy and therefore require regular 6–12-monthly endoscopic/biopsy surveillance. Early detection of malignant change is associated with improved survival from definitive surgery.

7.4 ANTRAL GASTRITIS AND PEPTIC ULCER DISEASE

The incidence and mortality from peptic ulcer disease (PUD) rises very significantly after the age of 60. The risk factors of PUD in old age are no different from those in younger people, except that the proportion of cases attributable to aspirin and other NSAID use is greater in the older group. Peptic ulcer resulting from NSAID usage is associated with increased mortality, since many of these cases will not have experienced major dyspepsia, due to the analgesic effects of the NSAID, and the first presentation may be with ulcer perforation or catastrophic haemorrhage. In one large UK study ibuprofen and diclofenac had the lowest risk, indomethacin, naproxen and piroxicam had intermediate risk, and azapropazone and ketoprofen had the highest risk of peptic ulcer bleeding. *Helicobacter pylori* infection rates rise steadily with advancing age, so that an estimated 70–80% of people over age 65 carry this organism in the gastric mucosa. Detection of *H. pylori* is also associated with acute and chronic antral gastritis (as distinct from autoimmune diffuse chronic gastritis, associated with pernicious anaemia). Endoscopy is recommended in older people with suspected gastritis/PUD, since it is the only reliable way to rapid diagnosis, detection of *H. pylori* (with urease testing indicated by colour change) and exclusion of gastric malignancy. Eradication of *H. pylori* in the presence of PUD is strongly recommended at any age, since the relapse of PUD with associated *H. pylori* infection is approximately 70%. Details of medical management of *H. pylori*-associated and NSAID-associated PUD are included in Table 7.2. Surgery is seldom required for PUD nowadays. However, operative intervention is still necessary in occasional cases of perforation, uncontrolled haemorrhage, gastric outlet obstruction and unremitting ulcer disease (despite prolonged high-dose proton pump inhibitor therapy, eradication of *H. pylori* and exclusion of NSAID usage).

Table 7.2   Management of peptic ulcer disease

(A) *Helicobacter pylori* DU
First detection: *H. pylori* eradication therapy, i.e. amoxycillin 1 g b.i.d. *plus* clarithromycin 500 mg b.i.d. *plus* omeprazole 20 mg b.i.d. for 1 week (eradication rate 89%), followed by ulcer healing therapy, i.e. H_2-antagonist or sucralfate for 4–8 weeks.
Relapse/refractory DU: Re-endoscope to look for persistent *H. pylori* and repeat previous therapy if detected. Long-term maintenance therapy with H_2-antagonist or proton pump inhibitor indicated following second relapse within 1 year.

(B) NSAID DU
Stop NSAID, recommend alternative non-NSAID analgesia. Treat ulcer with H_2-antagonist or sucralfate for 4–8 weeks. Eradicate *H. pylori* if detected.
Need to continue NSAID therapy: give continuous therapeutic doses of proton pump inhibitor or misoprostol 200 µg q.i.d. with NSAID.

(C) *H. pylori* GU
First detection: Multiple biopsies of margin of GU to exclude malignancy, followed by treatment as with *H. pylori* DU, but continue ulcer-healing therapy for 12 weeks. Repeat endoscopy after 12 weeks to ensure ulcer healing.
Relapsed/refractory GU: Exclude NSAID mucosal insult. Repeat biopsies of ulcer margin and re-check for *H. pylori*. Repeat *H. pylori* eradication if detected and use omeprazole 40 mg o.d. (or lansoprazole 60 mg o.d.) for 8 weeks. Long-term maintenance therapy with H_2-antagonist or proton pump inhibitor indicated following second relapse within 1 year.

(D) NSAID GU
As with NSAID DU, but biopsies of ulcer essential to exclude malignancy. If NSAID cannot be stopped, give omeprazole 20–40 mg o.d. (or lansoprazole 30–60 mg o.d.) until ulcer healed. Maintenance therapy with misoprostol 200 µg q.i.d. or proton pump inhibitors gives effective prophylaxis for NSAID GU if NSAID therapy must be continued.

DU, duodenal ulcer; GU, gastric ulcer; NSAID, non-steroidal anti-inflammatory drug; o.d., once daily; b.i.d., twice daily; q.i.d., four times daily.

7.5 INTESTINAL MALABSORPTION

The principal causes of intestinal malabsorption in older people are pancreatic exocrine insufficiency (usually following chronic pancreatitis), gluten enteropathy, previous gastric surgery and small intestinal bacterial overgrowth. Small bowel bacterial overgrowth may result from a variety of conditions, including large duodenal diverticula, jejunal diverticulosis, previous surgery (e.g. Billroth II partial gastrectomy, ileocaecal valve resection), small intestinal stricture or fistula and motility disorders (e.g. diabetic autonomic neuropathy, scleroderma). Although there is usually a structural abnormality associated with small bowel bacterial overgrowth, it has been shown to occur occasionally in the radiologically normal small intestine. Elderly people may present with symptoms of anaemia (folate, B_{12} deficiency), muscle weakness and falls (malnutrition), bone pain (osteomalacia), bruising (vitamin K deficiency), peripheral or optic neuropathy or myopathy (B_{12} deficiency), rather than with classical symptoms of steatorrhoea. Malabsorption should be suspected in patients with unexplained diarrhoea or who fail to gain weight despite documented high calorie intake. Useful investigations in suspected malabsorption are:

  (i) Microscopic examination of stool samples with Sudan III stain to detect fat droplets, indicating fat malabsorption.
 (ii) Five-hour urinary xylose excretion test. After ingestion of 25 g of D-xylose, urinary excretion should normally exceed 4.5 g and 1 hour blood levels should normally be >30 mg/dl. Lower levels indicate carbohydrate malabsorption.
(iii) Bentiromide test, which depends on a synthetic peptide being specifically cleaved by pancreatic chymotrysin, releasing para-aminobenzoic acid (PABA), which is measured in serum and urine. A normal test effectively excludes pancreatic exocrine insufficiency and about 80% of severe cases will have abnormal tests.
 (iv) Small intestinal biopsy obtained by endoscopy to detect villous atrophy consistent with gluten enteropathy.
  (v) Hydrogen breath testing after ingestion of 10 g of lactulose. Small bowel bacterial overgrowth will result in metabolism of lactulose with release of hydrogen, which is absorbed and excreted through the lungs. Detection of a rise of hydrogen by more than 10 p.p.m.

Table 7.3   Management of main causes of intestinal malabsorption in old age

---

(A) Pancreatic exocrine failure: supplemental pancreatic enzyme capsules (ensure at least 30 000 units of lipase with each meal), with or without acid suppression or as enteric-coated preparations, if insufficient therapeutic response.
(B) Gluten enteropathy: gluten-restricted diet (complete gluten restriction may be unmanageable for some elderly patients).
(C) Small bowel bacterial overgrowth (non-surgical causes): tetracycline 250 mg four times daily or metronidazole 200 mg twice daily for 7 days, repeated if necessary.

---

in the breath above baseline within 1–2 hours is consistent with bacterial fermentation of lactulose.

(vi) Imaging: plain X-rays will detect pancreatic calcification diagnostic of chronic pancreatitis and barium follow-through studies will detect abnormal motility patterns, blind loops, jejunal diverticulosis, small bowel mucosal thickening (infiltrative disease), and small bowel Crohn's disease.

Nutritional and vitamin deficiencies must be corrected in addition to treatment of underlying causes. Specific treatment of the principal causes of intestinal malabsorption in old people is detailed in Table 7.3.

7.6   MESENTERIC ISCHAEMIA

Although uncommon, mesenteric ischaemia syndromes are important, since they occur predominantly in old age and are often fatal if not detected early and, where appropriate, managed aggressively. Mesenteric ischaemia may be acute or chronic. **Acute small intestinal ischaemia** presents with sudden onset of abdominal pain, which progresses rapidly to peritonism and paralytic ileus. **Acute colonic ischaemia** may result in lower abdominal pain, fever and bloody diarrhoea. The patient usually has arteriopathy, often with a history of moderate or heavy melaena, and background atrial fibrillation, cardiac failure or valvular heart disease. Bruits may be detectable in the abdomen, in the neck and groins, and pedal pulses are often absent. Plain abdominal X-rays typically show ileus, mucosal 'thumb-printing' (oedema) and gas in the lining of the bowel. Neutrophil leucocytosis and metabolic acidosis are characteristic features, but are non-specific. The diagnostic test for acute mesenteric ischaemia is laparotomy, where the surgeon determines whether or not the ischaemic bowel is viable, and whether revascularization, resection of non-viable intestine or non-specific treatment is appropriate. Although younger patients with extensive small intestinal infarction may survive with a reasonably good quality of life with short bowel syndrome, provided they can tolerate chronic parenteral nutrition with a tunnelled feeding line sited in a large vein, this is seldom appropriate in elderly patients because of the risk of major complications and poor quality of life. Most cases of colonic ischaemia are single, self-limiting events without major sequelae, which resolve with supportive therapy only.

Chronic mesenteric ischaemia is often difficult to diagnose because of non-specific symptoms and findings on endoscopic and radiological investigation. Useful clues to the diagnosis are pain occurring after food in the absence of peptic ulcer, gallstone or pancreatic disease, and abdominal bruits. Chronic colonic ischaemia may present with colonic stricture, episodic bloody diarrhoea and non-specific ulceration on colonoscopy and biopsy. Mesenteric arteriography is the definitive investigation and may present the experienced vascular radiologist with an opportunity for revascularization by balloon angioplasty. If this fails, definitive bypass revascularization may be curative, but perioperative morbidity and mortality rates are significantly higher in elderly patients.

7.7 CONSTIPATION AND FAECAL INCONTINENCE

Constipation is a common and important symptom in older people. Although there is no convincing evidence of reduced bowel transit time in old age, age-related comorbidity and polypharmacy are the common causes of constipation. A detailed history, with particular emphasis on dietary fibre intake and drugs, is important to help identify the cause(s) of constipation. Recent change in bowel habit and weight loss or rectal bleeding are indications for urgent investigation to exclude colonic malignancy. Drugs are often the cause of constipation (Table 7.4) and details of all drugs taken (prescription and non-prescription) should be sought. Constipation is also associated with any cause of reduced physical activity (e.g. stroke, Parkinson's disease), metabolic disorders (e.g. diabetes mellitus, hypothyroidism, hypercalcaemia, hypokalaemia), depressive illness and chronic stimulant laxative abuse. Faecal impaction represents the extreme end of the constipation spectrum and may be associated with complications such as faecal incontinence, urinary retention with overflow incontinence, colonic obstruction, pressure ('stercoral') ulceration and perforation. Faecal incontinence results from constipation/faecal impaction in more than 90% of cases. In these circumstances, faecal incontinence is not usually due to reduced anal sphincter or reduced sphincter squeeze pressure but is caused by the combination of an obtuse anorectal angle, lower anal pressures and anal desensitization. Impaired anal sensation leads to impaired warning of impending faecal leakage so that voluntary anal sphincter contraction does not occur, resulting in incontinence.

When underlying causes or drugs have been excluded, treatment depends on the severity and duration of constipation. **Faecal impaction** should be managed by colonic disimpaction with regular enemas until there is no further response; this may take 7–10 days to achieve. **Phosphate enemas** which contain sodium acid phosphate draw water into the colon osmotically, increasing the water content of the faecal mass and causing rectal/colonic distension that triggers defecation. Sodium citrate-based enemas (e.g. Micralax) are alternatives, but should be used cautiously in patients with impaired sodium or water balance. If phosphate enemas fail, arachis or olive oil enemas may be tried. Where enemas and laxatives fail to induce defecation, powerful **saline osmotic laxative solutions** may be helpful, e.g. magnesium

Table 7.4 Drugs that commonly cause constipation

Opioid analgesics
Anticholinergics
● tricyclic antidepressants
● antispasmodics (e.g. oxybutinin)
● antiarrhythmics (e.g. disopyramide, procainamide)
● phenothiazines
● antihistamines
Calcium antagonists (particularly verapamil)
Loop diuretics
Iron
Aluminium-containing antacids
Antispasticity (e.g. baclofen)

sulphate 5–10 g in water, sodium picosulphate combined with magnesium citrate (Picolax) or polyethylene glycol.

Laxatives may be used to prevent recurrence of faecal impaction, particularly in frail elderly patients, until the underlying problem is resolved (if this is possible). Regular laxatives and weekly or twice weekly enemas may be necessary in immobile patients who are at high risk of recurrent impaction. There are four classes of laxatives:

(i) **Stimulant laxatives**—these act by a stimulant effect on the myenteric plexus which promotes colonic motility. Examples are **senna**, **danthron**, **bisacodyl**.

(ii) **Osmotic laxatives**—these act by retaining water in the intestinal lumen, thereby increasing the water content and bulk of faeces. Examples include magnesium sulphate, sodium picosulphate, polyethylene glycol and lactulose. **Lactulose** is the most widely prescribed osmotic laxative, and is a disaccharide comprising fructose and galactose. It is converted to lactic and acetic acids by fermenting colonic bacteria, which are not absorbed and therefore enhance colonic water content, which prevents stool hardening.

(iii) **Stool softeners**—these act by lubricating the stool surface either directly (e.g. liquid paraffin) or indirectly by lowering stool surface tension (e.g. **docusate sodium**, which has some stimulant properties also). Stool softeners used alone are not very effective in the management of constipation. However, they may be combined usefully with stimulant laxatives, as in codanthromer (danthron plus poloxamer) and codanthrusate (danthron plus docusate sodium).

(iv) **Bulk laxatives**—these are indigestible polysaccharides, normally found in plant fibre. The most widely used bulk laxative is **wheat bran**, which when taken in doses of 20–30 g daily with a fluid allowance of not less than 1500 ml, usually prevents constipation. Bran may be made more palatable if taken with prune juice, other fruit juice or mixed with yoghurt. Alternative bulk agents are **ispaghula husk** and **methylcellulose**, which may be mixed with drinks or foodstuffs. Bulk laxatives should be avoided until faecal impaction/constipation is completely resolved by other methods.

Once colonic faecal loading/impaction is resolved, relapse may be prevented by regular bowel evacuation using stimulant laxatives, of which senna is the cheapest and is as effective as other stimulant agents. The dose of senna is 15–30 mg nocte (2–4 tablets, calculated by content of sennoside B), which usually produces a desire to defecate within 8 hours. Increased dietary fibre may be introduced gradually over ensuing days and weeks, as senna is gradually withdrawn. Senna should not be used for more than a few weeks at a time, and certainly not as a continuous prescription. Senna at full dose may not be effective, particularly in patients with longstanding exposure to laxatives for chronic constipation, and there is little point in trying another stimulant laxative. Senna may be usefully combined with ispaghula (e.g. Manevac), which is more effective than lactulose and cheaper. However, lactulose may be tried as an alternative to stimulant laxatives, although it is not usually effective where senna has failed. In such cases, regular enemas once or twice weekly may be the only means of maintaining bowel clearance.

Resolution of faecal impaction/constipation cures most cases of faecal incontinence. However, some patients will suffer persisting soiling as a result of neurological damage to anal sphincter control (e.g. stroke, spinal cord disorders) or as a result of lack of awareness of a full rectum (e.g. dementia). In these cases, it may be possible to control bowel evacuation by using regular doses of constipating drugs (e.g. codeine phosphate) in tandem with twice weekly colonic evacuations with enemas.

7.8 COLONIC DIVERTICULAR DISEASE

Colonic diverticular disease is common in older people (40–50% of persons over 65) but is symptomatic in only a minority. Symptoms include recurrent colicky lower abdominal pain (usually associated with constipation), sometimes acute diverticulitis, occasionally diverticular abscess formation with fever, leucocytosis and localized abdominal tenderness, and rarely brisk rectal bleeding. Pulsion diverticula probably arise from increased intraluminal colonic pressure with powerful propulsive colonic contractions when there is persistent or recurring constipation. Diverticular disease is seldom seen in older people from countries where there is a high fibre content in the diet, and increasing dietary fibre helps prevent painful relapses in affected individuals. Bulk laxatives can be helpful if increasing dietary fibre is impractical or unpalatable. Non-steroidal anti-inflammatory drugs (e.g. diclofenac 25–50 mg three times a day orally or 75 mg intramuscularly) are preferred to opioids for pain relief. Pethidine may be necessary for severe pain, but morphine and diamorphine should be avoided if possible, because they are highly constipating and will ultimately exacerbate painful diverticular disease. Anticholinergic antispasmodics (e.g. mebeverine, dicyclomine) may be helpful for pain relief also, but tend to be less well tolerated in elderly than in younger patients.

Acute diverticulitis occurs when the mouth of a diverticulum becomes obstructed by a faecolith, causing stasis and infection within the diverticulum. The patient has localized pain and tenderness, usually accompanied by fever and leucocytosis, although these features may be absent in some elderly people, masking the diagnosis. Ultrasonic or CT imaging help confirm parabolic abscess formation and it may be possible to drain an abscess under radiological control. Acute diverticulitis is treated with **analgesics** (as for painful diverticular disease), **broad-spectrum intravenous antibiotics** (such as cefuroxime plus metronidazole) and **intravenous fluids** with 'nil by mouth'. Surgery is usually indicated if the patient's clinical status fails to improve after 72 hours. Where **surgery** is appropriate in acute diverticulitis, a two-stage procedure starting with resection of the diseased segment of colon and a diverting colostomy (Hartmann's procedure), followed some weeks later by secondary end-to-end anastomosis, is preferred. Large paracolic abscesses should be drained radiologically and antibiotic therapy given for 2–3 weeks before definitive surgery, if possible. Peritonitis requires emergency surgery in all cases, where appropriate. Perforated diverticular abscesses may result in fistulation into the bladder, vagina, ureter and ileum. Elective sigmoid colectomy and fistula closure is required in these cases. Rarely, erosion of a small artery at the mouth of a diverticulum may result in major haemorrhage. Fortunately, most of these cases settle with transfusion and conservative management. Clearly, rectal bleeding in these patients should not be ascribed to known diverticular disease until other causes have been excluded, particularly colon cancer.

7.9 ANTIBIOTIC-ASSOCIATED DIARRHOEA

Diarrhoea may be caused by virtually all antibiotics. The cause may be drug-specific (e.g. accelerated intestinal transit time with erythromycin) or may result from *Clostridium difficile* infection, as in about 20% of cases of antibiotic-associated diarrhoea. *Clostridium difficile* diarrhoea is an increasing problem in hospitals, nursing and residential homes since the 1980s. Other risk factors for *Clostridium difficile* diarrhoea include old age, physical frailty, enteral tube feeding and poor standards of hygiene among hospitalized patients. Colonization with *Clostridium difficile* occurs in 3% of the healthy adult population, but hospital admission increased the colonization rate to 21% in one study, where the median hospital stay was 12 days. Patients who are colonized but do not have diarrhoea do not appear to be a risk to other patients. Symptoms usually occur 4–7 days after starting antibiotic therapy, and may range in severity from occasional watery diarrhoea which resolves within 24–48 hours of stopping the antibiotic, to severe, life-threatening pseudomembranous colitis that sometimes progresses to toxic megacolon or perforation and death. The mechanism of *Clostridium difficile* diarrhoea is the production of toxins (A and B) which have a direct cytotoxic effect on colonic mucosa. The diagnosis is made by detection of *Clostridium difficile* toxin in stool samples, which is a quick, highly specific and cheap test.

In former years, clindamycin was the antibiotic most commonly associated with *Clostridium difficile* diarrhoea, but its use is now restricted. Nowadays, the most commonly implicated antibiotics are **amoxycillin**,

Table 7.5   Management of *Clostridium difficile* diarrhoea

(1) Stop the offending antibiotic. Give an alternative antibiotic less likely to cause *C. difficile* diarrhoea (e.g. benzylpenicillin, quinolone, aminoglycoside) if continuing antibiotic therapy is necessary for the primary infection.
(2) Isolate the patient.
(3) Institute strict hygiene measures among all attending staff.
(4) For mild cases, observe and treat expectantly. For moderate severity cases, give oral metronidazole 800 mg immediately followed by 400 mg three times daily for 7 days. In severe cases (i.e. full-blown pseudomembranous colitis), oral vancomycin 125 mg four times daily for 7–10 days with full resuscitative measures is recommended.

cephalosporins and **ciprofloxacin**. The management of *Clostridium difficile* diarrhoea is detailed in Table 7.5. Some 10–20% of cases relapse within 1–3 weeks of stopping treatment and repeat courses of metronidazole or vancomycin may be required (metronidazole is considerably cheaper). Occasionally, recurrent relapse is a problem despite repeat courses of anti-*Clostridium difficile* therapy. In such cases, a slowly tapered dose of vancomycin or cholestyramine (which binds and inactivates the *Clostridium difficile* toxin) may be tried, although firm evidence to support this approach is lacking.

FURTHER READING

Anonymous. Malnourished inpatients: overlooked and undertreated. *Drug Ther Bull* 1996; 34:57–60.

Langman MJS, Weil J, Wainwright P et al. Risks of bleeding peptic ulcer associated with individual non-steroidal anti-inflammatory drugs. *Lancet* 1994; 343:1075–1078.

McWhirter JP, Pennington CR. Incidence and recognition of malnutrition in hospital. *Br Med J* 1994; 308:945–948.

Settle CD. *Clostridium difficile*. *Br J Hosp Med* 1996; 56:398–400.

Tobin GW. *Incontinence in the Elderly*. Edward Arnold, London, 1992, pp 86–91.

Chapter 8

Rheumatological Disorders

8.1 OSTEOARTHRITIS

Osteoarthritis (OA) is the most commonly encountered arthropathy in elderly people. Pathologically it is a condition of synovial joints characterized by focal cartilage loss and accompanying bone and cartilage repair at the joint margin. Clinical symptoms are usually local and involve the distal interphalangeal joints (Heberden's nodes), proximal interphalangeal joints, base of thumb, knees and hip joints. In general, clinical symptoms correlate with radiographic findings except for spinal disease where there is often a discordance between radiographic change and clinical features. Cervical myelopathy or cauda equina syndrome from degenerative spinal canal stenosis may manifest primarily with gait weakness or sphincter disorders.

Pain in early OA is related to the use of the joint and is mechanical in nature. Rest or nocturnal pain occurs late in the disease. Joint stiffness occurs after rest but usually improves within a few minutes of activity. The initial approach to the patient with OA is to determine whether the symptoms are coming from the joint itself, which should be examined for tenderness, reduced range of movement, crepitus and deformity. Swelling or joint enlargement may be bony or due to synovial tissue with or without effusion. Radiologically, there may be evidence of cartilage loss with joint space narrowing and the presence of osteophytes and sclerosis. If an effusion is present and an inflammatory reaction or infection is suspected the joint should be aspirated and the fluid sent for Gram stain, culture and microscopic examination for crystals.

8.1.1 Treatment

The aims of treatment are patient education, pain relief, optimization of function and minimization of progression. Many patients with OA benefit from a simple explanation of the illness and should be questioned about the effect of symptoms on daily activity. Beneficial lifestyle changes are detailed in Table 8.1. Drug treatment is aimed at symptom control. Disease progression is not inevitable but a slow progression is likely. Surgery is reserved for advanced disease when patients are severely limited in performing everyday tasks due to pain or skeletal deformity. Rehabilitation is therefore the mainstay of treatment for patients with mild to moderate disease. Patients should be encouraged to maintain daily activities within the limits of their pain and those with hip and/or knee OA are prescribed individualized exercise programmes with the aim of improving muscle strength, reducing joint contractures and increasing the range of motion. The load on weight-bearing joints can be reduced by use of a cane in the opposite hand. Superficial heat and ice are also important.

8.1.2 Pain Control

Adequate doses of analgesics such as paracetamol given regularly provide adequate pain relief for most patients. In healthy patients no more than 4 g per day should be given and in patients with mild liver disease the dose should be halved. Moderate-potency opioids such as codeine may also be used sparingly. If there is superimposed inflammation, or if paracetamol is ineffective, a non-steroidal anti-inflammatory

Table 8.1   Changes in lifestyle for patients with osteoarthritis

General
Maintain optimal weight
Regular exercise

Specific
Strengthening of local muscles
Appropriate footwear, e.g. insoles to counteract knee varus; trainers
Walking aids, e.g. patella femoral strapping; walking sticks

agent (NSAID) may be more appropriate although there is concern about the increase in use of these agents in elderly patients. NSAIDs work by inhibiting the enzyme cyclo-oxygenase (COX), which is responsible for the production of prostaglandins from arachidonic acid. Recent studies have shown that there are two isoenzymes of COX: constitutive COX-1, responsible for the production of prostaglandins which protect the gastric mucosa and maintain renal blood flow, and inducible COX-2, responsible for production of prostaglandins which drive the inflammatory response. Some NSAIDs such as indomethacin may accelerate the clinical progression of OA and NSAIDs often cause gastrointestinal symptoms with an increased risk of bleeding and perforation from peptic ulcer disease. Patients with even mildly impaired renal function starting an NSAID may suffer an abrupt deterioration in renal function and hyperkalaemia. Idiopathic hepatotoxicity may also occur. Although some agents are advertised as having fewer side-effects all are potentially capable of causing gastrointestinal bleeding and renal failure in elderly patients.

NSAIDs should be avoided in this age group but may provide very effective pain relief in those with an inflammatory component or inadequate symptom control, if they are used. Patients should be maintained on the lowest dose possible to achieve the desired effect. **Ibuprofen** is the safest NSAID when used in low doses (200 mg three times daily). Newer, more COX-2 selective NSAIDs such as **meloxicam** appear to have an equivalent efficacy to standard NSAIDs with fewer gastrointestinal side-effects and may be appropriate in high risk patients, but the data is still very limited. **Nabumetone** may be less likely to cause renal problems. Symptoms of osteoarthritis are often episodic and the requirement for NSAIDs should be regularly re-evaluated. Patients at high risk of gastrointestinal toxicity, e.g. the frail elderly over 75 years, or those with a past history of peptic ulcer, benefit from the concurrent administration of **misoprostol**, which may be combined with an NSAID. However, diarrhoea and abdominal pain occur commonly with miso-prostol and recent data show that proton pump inhibitors are the drugs of first choice in the prevention and healing of NSAID-induced gastric and duodenal ulcers. Compliance tends to be good because of lack of toxicity and once daily dosing. Topical NSAIDs (e.g. **piroxicam**, **ketoprofen** or **diclofenac**) have similar efficacy to oral preparations in patients with OA but have fewer adverse effects. They are indicated for patients with just a few symptomatic, easily accessible joints.

Inflammatory flare of OA is not uncommon and it may sometimes be associated with evidence of calcium pyrophosphate crystals with chondrocalcinosis on X-ray (see section 8.4). Occasional corticosteroid injections (two to three per year) in the elderly for OA of the knee often works very well to reduce pain and increase mobility and is probably much safer than NSAIDs or surgery. Corticosteroid injections are also useful in patients with moderate OA in whom NSAIDs are contraindicated, e.g. patients taking warfarin or with renal disease.

8.2 RHEUMATOID ARTHRITIS

Rheumatoid arthritis (RA) is a chronic systemic inflammatory disease affecting approximately 1% of the world's population. Disease patterns vary and the rheumatoid factor will be negative in at least 30% of patients, especially early in the disease. RA may be manifested clinically by malaise and fatigue, followed by joint inflammation which may involve the wrists, metacarpal phalangeal joints, proximal interphalangeal joints, elbows, shoulders, cervical spine, hips, knees, ankles and metatarsal phalangeal joints. Affected joints are painful and stiff, particularly in the morning and after periods of activity. Affected joints may be swollen, warm and tender. Joint effusions, palpable synovial hypertrophy and rheumatoid nodules at pressure points (e.g. at elbows, Achilles tendon) may be present. Laboratory findings may include a mild anaemia of chronic disease and a raised erythrocyte sedimentation rate (ESR) in addition to a positive rheumatoid factor. Synovial fluid analysis of inflamed joints reveals a raised white cell count with 50% or more neutrophils. X-rays of affected joints may show bony erosions, periarticular osteopenia and joint space narrowing. Older patients who have had longstanding RA are likely to have accumulated joint deformities which make them more likely to fall. In addition, they may have significant osteoporosis, particularly if steroids have been used, which increases their risk for fractures. RA developing over the age of 60 can be clinically similar to polymyalgia rheumatica. Low-dose glucocorticoids used as sole therapy may provide very effective symptom control and improve function in elderly patients with a limited lifespan. Extra-articular manifestations of rheumatoid arthritis are similar to those in younger patients (Table 8.2).

Table 8.2 Extra-articular manifestations of rheumatoid arthritis

Vasculitis	
Pulmonary	Pleural effusion
	Fibrosing alveolitis
	Nodules
Cardiac	Pericarditis
	Conduction defects
Skin	Palmar erythema
	Cutaneous vasculitis
	Pyoderma gangrenosum
Eyes	Sjögren's syndrome
	Episcleritis
	Scleritis
Neurological	Peripheral nerve entrapment
	Mononeuritis multiplex
	Peripheral neuropathy
	Cervical cord compression

8.2.1 Physical Treatment

Physiotherapy plays a key role in the treatment of RA and local measures such as heat and cold may reduce pain and form part of a rehabilitation programme of exercise to improve muscle strength and joint mobility. The aims of occupational therapy are to educate patients to protect joints and improve function by provision of appropriate aids and appliances. Surgery may be necessary to relieve pain and restore function in those with advanced secondary OA.

8.2.2 Pharmacological Treatment

Paracetamol should be used for simple pain relief. NSAIDs can provide symptomatic relief but do not modify the course of the disease (see above). Although ibuprofen should be tried first in elderly patients, stronger agents such as slow-release diclofenac 75 mg daily may be needed. Intra-articular corticosteroids may provide short-term symptomatic relief. Long-acting depot drugs are best (see section 8.7). Triamcinolone is used for large joints. Methylprednisolone is preferable for superficial joints and tendon sheaths because of the lower incidence of subcutaneous and skin atrophy. The use of oral corticosteroids in RA remains controversial because of fears of adverse effects such as osteoporosis. However, long-term low-dose oral corticosteroids are often used in elderly patients with significant functional difficulty.

Table 8.3 Disease-modifying drugs in rheumatoid arthritis

Drug	Adverse effects	Effectiveness	Monitoring
Hydroxy-chloroquine	Retinopathy (rare)	Used for milder RA, e.g. mono/oligo-articular, seronegative	Ophthalmic
Sulphasalazine	Nausea Rash Bone marrow toxicity Hepatitis Transient oligospermia	Popular first choice, especially for moderate RA	FBC, LFTs
Penicillamine	Metallic taste Nausea Rash Bone marrow toxicity Proteinuria	Can cause remission but toxic	FBC, urine
Gold	Rash Proteinuria Bone marrow toxicity Diarrhoea (oral gold)	Can cause remission but toxic	FBC, urine
Azathioprine	Nausea Hepatitis Bone marrow toxicity Risk of lymphoma and skin cancer	Used for synovitis and systemic complications	FBC, LFTs
Methotrexate	Nausea Bone marrow toxicity Alveolitis Hepatic fibrosis Folate deficiency	Drug of first choice for severe RA	FBC, LFTs
Cyclosporin	Renal impairment Hypertension	Use in resistant RA	BP, creatinine

FBC, full blood count; LFTs, liver function tests; BP, blood pressure.

Short courses of steroids may be useful as 'bridge' therapy while second-line agents are being introduced.

Second-line drugs may alter the course of RA (Table 8.3). Indications for their use in elderly patients are similar to those in younger patients but the elderly may be at higher risk of adverse reactions, especially with cytotoxic agents. Appropriate caution and patient selection are necessary.

8.3 GOUT

Gout is caused by intra-articular deposits of urate. As with pseudogout (see section 8.4), the disorder may appear after many years of silent deposition of crystals, so elderly people experience the worst symptoms. Acute gouty arthritis in elderly patients differs from gout in younger adults in several other respects. Women are affected almost as often as men and polyarticular attacks are common. Fever and delirium may also occur. In addition, urate renal calculi are less likely. The increased frequency of gout in postmenopausal women seems to be due to loss of oestrogen-promoted uricosuria and long-term use of thiazides and loop diuretics. The diagnosis is usually obvious clinically and patients present with attacks of severe joint pain which affect characteristic sites and subside over 3–10 days even without treatment. Acute gout is often associated with local cellulitis and may causes a bursitis, e.g. olecranon. The diagnosis is supported by a raised plasma urate concentration, but if not, aspiration of an affected joint to determine the presence of intracellular negatively birefringent crystals is definitive.

8.3.1 Treatment

Acute attacks of gout can be treated with **NSAIDs** or **colchicine**. Although NSAIDs have a high risk of toxicity in elderly patients, a short course of indomethacin or diclofenac is an appropriate and effective treatment for acute gout. Colchicine is often preferred and a dose of 1 mg is followed by 500 µg every 2 to 3 hours until relief of pain occurs. No more than 4 mg should be given in total. At higher doses significant toxicity occurs and includes nausea, vomiting, profuse diarrhoea, rashes, nephritis and hepatitis. Corticosteroids are indicated for patients in whom colchicine or NSAIDs are contraindicated or for unusual attacks refractory to conventional treatment. Prednisolone/ prednisone 40–60 mg should be given until a response appears, then tapered rapidly. Intra-articular steroids are very effective for large joint gout that fails to settle with conventional treatment.

The decision to begin allopurinol is more difficult in the elderly. Occasional attacks may be treated symptomatically and in some patients changing from thiazides to an alternative antihypertensive may prevent further attacks. Lifestyle changes are also important and include weight loss and reduction of alcohol intake. Prophylaxis should be considered if the patient suffers recurrent attacks despite these measures. Allopurinol is a highly effective hypouricaemic agent but may be associated with toxic effects in the first few weeks of therapy which comprise fever, rash, eosinophilia, hepatic and renal impairment. Toxicity is more common in elderly patients and has a reported mortality rate of 25%. For this reason the starting dose should be reduced to 100 to 150 mg per day in elderly patients and increased slowly. A dose sufficient to keep the serum urate <350 µmol/l is required, although in general this will be lower than in younger people because of the age-related decline in renal function. To prevent acute attacks of gout during initiation of allopurinol colchicine 500 µg twice daily should be given until a month after the hyperuricaemia is corrected.

8.4 PSEUDOGOUT

The term pseudogout describes an acute inflammatory synovitis induced by shedding of calcium pyrophosphate crystals in the joints and chondrocalcinosis describes the radiographic appearance of calcified joint cartilage. Chrondrocalcinosis is found in 50% of individuals by the ninth decade of life. Rarely pseudogout may be associated with hyperparathyroidism, hypothyroidism, hypomagnesaemia and haemochromatosis. Attacks of acute monoarthritis affecting the knee and wrist are typical. The aspirate from an involved joint will show positively birefringent crystals in neutrophils. Most patients have radiological evidence of calcification in the knee menisci and other cartilages.

Chondrocalcinosis occurs frequently in OA and may result in attacks of pseudogout.

8.4.1 Treatment

Acute mono-articular attacks respond well to aspiration and steroid injection. An NSAID may be necessary in addition. Alternatively, colchicine may be used as in gout.

8.5 APATITE DISEASE

Deposition of apatite or hydroxyapatite crystals is associated with calcific periarthritis, tendonitis and joint disease such as the Milwaukee shoulder syndrome. The latter is a severe shoulder arthropathy of elderly women associated with shoulder instability, large, often bloody effusions and a previous history of trauma or renal disease. Rotator cuff tears and advanced joint degeneration are common and prognosis for recovering movement is poor. An episodic oligoarthritis may also occur with apatite disease, which should be suspected when crystals are absent from the synovial fluid and radiographs show articular and periarticular calcium deposits. Erosive arthritis may be seen, particularly in the shoulder.

8.6 SOFT TISSUE RHEUMATISM

Inflammation of periarticular soft tissue structures may result from trauma induced by strain or direct injury and from various rheumatic processes such as RA and gout. Common sites of inflammation include the shoulder (supraspinatus or bicipital head tendonitis), elbow (epicondylitis—tennis elbow), thumb (de Quervain's disease), hip (trochanter bursitis), knee (prepatellar bursitis) and heel (Achilles or calcaneal bursitis). Although pain and incapacity in these conditions may persist for many months they are usually self-limiting and the part played by inflammation is often unclear. Rest and immobilization provide adequate relief for most patients and are essential when weight-bearing tendons are involved. An NSAID may also be needed and physiotherapy will reduce pain and strengthen involved muscles to reduce the risk of recurrence. Randomized controlled studies of corticosteroid injections are few. Some have shown substantial benefit, for instance, from methylprednisolone injection for trigger finger and thumb and for a range of painful foot conditions. However, the results for painful shoulder and tennis elbow have been inconclusive.

8.7   ARTICULAR AND PERIARTICULAR CORTICOSTEROID INJECTIONS

Seven corticosteroids are available for intra-articular injections but only triamcinolone and methylprednisolone are used regularly. The dose injected (either alone or mixed with local anaesthetic) is determined by joint size, severity of pain and previous response. Smaller doses may be given into tendon sheaths and bursae or infiltrated around inflamed ligaments or tendons. Injection of corticosteroid into a joint aims to achieve a sustained concentration of the drug in the synovium and synovial fluid whilst minimizing plasma concentrations and the risk of systemic side-effects. After injection the corticosteroid is taken up by the synovial cells, then gradually absorbed into the blood and cleared.

Unwanted systemic effects appear rare after a single intra-articular injection but symptomatic hyperglycaemia may occur in diabetic patients and some suppression of the hypothalamic–pituitary–adrenal axis may occur. Unwanted local effects include iatrogenic septic arthritis or periarthritis and are most likely to occur in patients with rheumatoid arthritis on immunosuppressive therapy. Scrupulous skin cleansing and a 'no touch' technique are vital to avoid this complication, which may take up to 12 weeks to emerge after injection. Other unwanted effects include progressive damage to the joint from repeated intra-articular injections, soft tissue atrophy from periarticular injections and damage to tendons or nerves. The risk of tendon rupture is greatest for the Achilles tendon and long head of biceps tendon and every attempt should be made to avoid direct injection into a tendon.

8.8 OSTEOPOROSIS

Postmenopausal osteoporosis is a common disorder characterized by an increase in bone resorption relative to bone formation resulting in reduced bone mass and an increased risk of fractures. The three most common sites at which osteoporotic fractures appear are the spine, the femoral neck and the radius. The most important endogenous risk factors for osteoporosis are advanced age, female sex and Caucasian or Asian race. In women oestrogen deficiency is pivotal and conditions that lead to a premenopausal deficiency of oestrogen are strongly associated with the development of osteoporosis. These include early menopause or premenopausal oophorectomy, chronic illness, malabsorption and long-term corticosteroid therapy. Bone mass is also affected adversely by excessive alcohol, cigarette smoking and physical inactivity. Although calcium supplementation reduces age-related loss of bone mass a convincing reduction in fracture rates has not been demonstrated. Vitamin D deficiency may lead to secondary hyperparathyroidism with a consequent increase in cortical bone loss. Finally, low body mass index is a risk factor for and obesity protects against osteoporosis.

The clinical manifestations of osteoporosis appear late in the course of the disease when treatment is unsatisfactory. Therefore preventive treatment should be aimed at those at greatest risk. Patients usually present with fractures, particularly wedge or crush fractures of the spine. In at least a third of patients there is sudden severe back pain at the level of the fracture. Spinal cord compression is seldom associated with osteoporotic vertebral fractures and the presence of neurological signs is more suggestive of bony metastases or Paget's disease.

Conventional biochemical tests are usually normal in osteoporosis although alkaline phosphatase may be elevated immediately after the fracture has occurred. Lateral X-rays of the lumbar and dorsal spine will demonstrate fractures and osteopenia although the latter is a highly subjective radiological sign. Specific measurement of bone density is necessary to diagnose osteoporosis.

8.8.1   Treatment

Hormone replacement therapy (HRT, see Chapter 6), is the current regimen of choice for the prevention and treatment of osteoporosis in postmenopausal women. It reduces fracture risk in the spine and hip and may increase in bone mass. Some alternatives are available for women who cannot have HRT.

Bisphosphonates inhibit bone resorption and have been shown to increase the bone mass in spine, hip and total body and to reduce vertebral fractures when taken for 3 years. At present they are still being evaluated but they represent an alternative for postmenopausal osteo-porosis in women who are unable to tolerate HRT. The regimen currently used in the UK consists of repeated cycles of a 2 week course of etidronate 400 mg nocte followed by 11 weeks of elemental calcium at a dose of 500 mg/day. The etidronate should not be taken within 2 hours of eating because absorption is impaired by food. Nausea, constipation or diarrhoea sometimes occur. An alternative is continuous alendronic acid at a dose of 10 mg/day. Severe oesophageal problems have been reported including ulcers and erosions so the drug should be taken 30 minutes before breakfast with a glass of water and the patient should stand or sit upright for at least 30 minutes.

Calcitonin inhibits bone resorption by a direct action on the osteoclast which has calcitonin receptors. It has been shown to reduce or prevent menopausal bone loss but there is no evidence that it reduces fracture rates. It is administered subcutaneously or by intra-nasal insufflation. Salmon calcitonin (salcatonin) is the most widely used. It has significant analgesic properties and may be effective in the treatment of bone pain associated with vertebral fracture, particularly in the acute phase. The dose is 50–100 IU daily until symptomatic relief has been obtained. Adverse effects include nausea, vomiting, flushing, diarrhoea, unpleas-ant taste in the mouth and pain at the injection site. These are minimized by giving the injection subcutaneously at night.

A **calcium** intake of 1 to 1.5 g is recommended in postmenopausal women and may need to be provided by supplements. Gentle **weight-bearing exercise** may be beneficial. **Vitamin D** supplements also have an important place and have been shown to reduce hip fractures, especially in the institutionalized elderly. A good option in elderly women is a combination tablet such as Calcichew D3 Forte, which combines 500 mg of elemental calcium with 400 units of cholecalciferol.

8.9   OSTEOMALACIA

In elderly patients osteomalacia is usually caused by a deficiency of vitamin D. The major source of vitamin D is from ultraviolet light in the sun converting 7-dehydrocholesterol in the skin to cholecalciferol. Dietary sources of vitamin D include fish, cereals and margarine. Cholecalciferol is hydroxylated in the liver and then the kidney to form the active metabolite 1,25-dihydroxycholecalciferol. The prevalence of osteomalacia in the elderly population is not known but it may affect up to 50% of unselected acute admissions to geriatric units. There are several reasons for this high prevalence in older people including decreased exposure to sunlight, poor diet and age-related decrease in the rate of hydroxylation of the parent compound to its active metabolite. Other mechanisms that may be important are gastrointestinal malabsorption of vitamin D which has been observed in sick old people, impaired hepatic hydroxylation and finally impaired renal hydroxylation if there is coexistent renal failure.

The classical symptoms of osteomalacia of bone pain and tenderness, fractures and proximal myopathy are rarely seen in the elderly or, if present, are attributed to other pathology. Bone pain tends to be diffuse and affects the ribs, spine and femora. The muscle weakness is associated with wasting and hypotonia. Fractures may occur following minimal trauma and are particularly common in the ribs. In severe longstanding osteomalacia, Looser's zones or pseudofractures may form in the ribs, pubic rami, scapulae and upper ends of the femora. They consist of a translucent band of demineralized bone resulting from an unhealed cortical microfracture. They may lead to subtrochanteric femoral neck fractures. Biochemical features include a raised serum alkaline phosphatase, a low normal corrected calcium and a low normal phosphate with otherwise normal liver function tests. These tests, however, are less specific in the elderly. In difficult cases bone biopsy may be helpful.

8.9.1 Treatment

Nutritional osteomalacia is best treated with ergocalciferol 30 µg (1200 IU) daily in the form of calcium and ergocalciferol tablets three daily. If compliance is a problem or if malabsorption is suspected, 600 000 IU of calciferol in oil can be given intramuscularly each year. Vitamin D deficiency caused by intestinal malabsorption or chronic liver disease usually requires up to 40 000 units of calciferol daily. For treatment of vitamin D deficiency due to renal disease see Chapter 10.

8.10 POLYMYALGIA RHEUMATICA AND GIANT CELL ARTERITIS

Polymyalgia rheumatica (PMR) is a syndrome characterized by pain and morning stiffness in the neck, shoulder girdle and pelvic girdle and is commonly associated with constitutional symptoms such as malaise and fatigue. The most useful clue to diagnosis is the abrupt onset and the symmetry of the symptoms. It may occur separately or in association with giant cell arteritis (GCA). Up to 90% of patients are over 60. In PMR the ESR is usually quite elevated. A mild normochromic normocytic anaemia is often present. Giant cell arteritis is a vasculitis that mainly involves the carotid and vertebrobasilar arteries and their branches. Symptoms include headache, jaw claudication, visual disturbances, scalp tenderness, decreased temporal artery pulse and constitutional symptoms. Sudden, irreversible visual loss may occur. Thoracic aortic aneurysm or dissection is an occasional complication. An ESR of over 100 mm in the first hour is common. Temporal artery biopsy of at least 2 cm in length should be obtained to make the diagnosis. When vision-related symptoms are present, corticosteroids should be started immediately and the biopsy arranged within a week.

8.10.1 Treatment

In PMR low doses of corticosteroids (prednisolone/prednisone 15 mg/day) often relieve symptoms within 1 week. Once symptoms have resolved and the ESR has normalized the steroids should be reduced by 2.5 mg every 2–4 weeks until 10 mg/day is reached. The dose should then be reduced by 1 mg every 2–6 weeks, relying on the presence and recurrence of typical symptoms to guide therapy. The aim of maintenance treatment is to prevent a relapse using the lowest possible dose of corticosteroids. ESR and C-reactive protein are unreliable in judging relapse. Higher doses of corticosteroids are needed to treat GCA. Starting doses of at least 40 mg are sufficient except in those with ocular symptoms in whom doses of up to 80 mg/day may be needed. Most patients will need treatment for at least 2 years but should be able to stop steroids after 3 to 5 years. Monitoring for relapse should continue for at least up to 1 year after stopping treatment. From 20% to 50% of patients may experience serious side-effects on the higher doses of steroids. Etidronate and calcium carbonate may be appropriate to prevent osteoporosis in women taking high doses of steroids for a prolonged period. This should be started early in elderly women at high risk since steroid-induced bone loss is most marked during the first 6 months of treatment.

8.11 PAGET'S DISEASE

Paget's disease may affect up to 10% of elderly people and is usually asymptomatic. It is a chronic disorder characterized by accelerated resorption and production of bone resulting in deformity and fragility. Osteoclastic bone resorption seen on radiographs as localized osteolytic areas (e.g. in the skull) occurs in the early phase of the disease. Later, increased osteoblastic activity occurs with formation of disorganized bone which lacks the normal trabecular pattern and is much weaker.

8.11.1 Clinical Features

Pain is the most common presenting feature and is typically deep, constant and worse at rest and at night. Pain may arise from increased vascularity, from distortion of the periosteum due to disorganized remodelling or from a focus of mechanical stress. It may arise in any affected bone but may also occur in adjacent joints which are damaged by weight bearing of deformed bones causing secondary osteoarthritis, particularly in the hip and knee.

The most frequent abnormality is bowing of the long bones, which occurs laterally in the femur and anteriorly in the tibia. Anterior bossing of the skull is also common. Expansion of the upper and lower jaw can cause dental malocclusion. Up to 15% of patients may sustain pathological fractures in abnormal bone. Fissure fractures occur in the long bones, especially the femur, tibia and humerus, and may be asymptomatic or painful. Complete fractures may also occur following minimal trauma. When these occur in the femur, subtrochanteric and shaft fractures are more common than femoral neck fractures which are seen in osteoporosis. Complete fracture in Paget's disease may be indicative of underlying sarcoma, particularly in the humerus. Although most fractures heal well with closed or surgical reduction the incidence of non-union may be 40%. Finally, vertebral body compression fractures are common. They may result in entrapment of the spinal cord leading rarely to quadriparesis or paraparesis.

Some of the neurological sequelae of Paget's disease result from invagination of the skull base (platybasia) caused by bone softening. Pressure on the brainstem precipitates ataxia, weakness with long tract compression, respiratory and vertebrobasilar insufficiency and cerebellar syndromes. Paget's disease of the skull may cause deafness in up to 50% of patients which may be either sensorineural, conductive or both. Narrowing of the optic foramen may produce papilloedema and optic atrophy but blindness is rare. Similarly, trigeminal neuralgia, facial palsy and bulbar palsy with dysphagia are occasionally seen in Paget's disease.

Osteosarcoma is a rare complication in Paget's disease affecting the pelvis and femur most commonly. The diagnosis should be considered in a previously stable patient who develops intense pain in an affected bone with a progressive lytic lesion and a rising alkaline phosphatase. The prognosis is poor with only 10% 5-year survival.

8.11.2   Diagnosis

The diagnosis is based primarily on the characteristic radiographic changes and raised alkaline phosphatase. Increased osteoclastic activity may be assessed by a 24-hour urinary hydroxyproline excretion or a spot fasting urine hydroxyproline/creatinine ratio, where available.

Radiological investigation may reveal characteristic lesions in affected bones with bony enlargement and cortical thickening. Bowing deformities in long bones and osteoarthritis in knees and hips are frequently seen. Osteolytic activity without an obvious adjacent sclerotic response may be seen in the osteoporosis circumscripta of the skull or the flame-shaped advancing front of a long bone. A characteristic appearance that differentiates Paget's from other conditions is the increased diameter of affected bones, particularly the spine and shafts of long bones. Isotope bone scan may also be indicated to identify the number and extent of Pagetic bone lesions.

8.11.3 Treatment

Previously, the only indication for specific treatment of Paget's disease was pain. More recently the trend is towards early aggressive treatment with the intention of modifying the natural history of the disease and preventing complications. Pagetic and related osteoarthritic pain may be reduced by simple analgesics and NSAIDs. Physiotherapy improves muscle function and maintains mobility. Correcting differences in leg length with shoe raises can sometimes abolish knee or hip pain without recourse to drugs. The indications for anti-Pagetic drugs are listed in Table 8.4.

All **bisphosphonates** are effective for Pagetic pain and disease activity and the sustained control of disease activity which they produce has

Table 8.4 Indications for treatment in Paget's disease

Pain arising from a known site of Paget's disease
Early potentially deforming disease
Osteolytic lesions, especially in weight-bearing joints
Skull involvement
Complications
  Progressive neurological syndromes
  Fissure fractures
  Immobilization hypercalcaemia
  High output cardiac failure
Increase in serum alkaline phosphatase or urinary hydroxyproline to twice maximum normal

resulted in their replacing calcitonin as drug of first choice. The aim should be to reduce serum alkaline phosphatase to normal. Etidronate, pamidronate and tiludronate are currently licensed for use in Paget's disease in the UK. Etidronate is given by mouth at 5 mg/kg/day for 6 months or 10 mg/kg/day for 3 months. It achieves good clinical response in about 50% of treated patients. The limiting factor is the risk of demineralization which can increase the risk of pathological fracture through Pagetic long bones. This is less likely to occur with the newer bisphosphonates. Pamidronate (ideally given in the day hospital) is administered by intravenous infusion at a dose of 30 mg weekly for 6 weeks. Bone turnover will be reduced by 60–70% and remission may be prolonged. A treatment course may be repeated every 6 months.

The use of **calcitonin** has largely been superseded by bisphosphonates but it may occasionally be needed to reduce bone blood flow before operation or bone pain following pathological fracture.

Paget's disease is generally considered to be in remission until bone turnover has increased by more than 25% above the minimum achieved after treatment as manifested by serum alkaline phosphatase.

8.12   SEPTIC ARTHRITIS

Acute infectious arthritis commonly occurs in older patients with previous joint damage. The infecting organisms are *Staphylococcus aureus* (70%) or *Streptococcus* species. Gram-negative organisms are less common except postoperatively or in the setting of neutropenia or urinary tract infection. The joint should be aspirated and synovial fluid sent for Gram's stain and culture and a differential white cell count. Blood cultures should also be sent. Intravenous antibiotics should be given for at least 4 weeks followed by oral antibiotics for a further 2 weeks or more, depending on response. *Staphylococcus aureus* should be treated with intravenous flucloxacillin 1 g four times daily combined with oral sodium fusidate 500 mg three times daily; *Streptococcus* with intravenous benzylpenicillin 1.2 mg 4-hourly; Gram-negative organisms with intravenous cefuroxime 1.5 g three times daily.

8.13 OSTEOMYELITIS

Osteomyelitis should be considered in patients with localized bone pain who are febrile or systemically unwell. The diagnosis is made by culturing the pathogen from bone or blood. Early bone biopsy and culture of tissue may be necessary to establish a diagnosis. The radiographic changes of soft tissue swelling, periosteal elevation, bone lysis, and sclerosis may lag several weeks behind the clinical presentation. Conditions that predispose to osteomyelitis are listed in Table 8.5. Osteomyelitis is most frequently caused by *Staphylococcus aureus*. Recurrent urinary tract infection may lead to vertebral osteomyelitis with Gram-negative bacilli. Osteomyelitis can usually be treated successfully by antimicrobial therapy but in the presence of a foreign body or vascular insufficiency surgical intervention may be necessary.

8.14 CARPAL TUNNEL SYNDROME

Paraesthesia, burning or numbness in the hand is often due to compression of the median nerve or carpal tunnel syndrome. Symptoms are worse at night and are relieved by shaking the hand/arm. Motor dysfunction and ultimately thenar wasting occurs. It may be secondary to lesions within or around the wrist joint such as a ganglion or wrist synovitis. It may also be associated with rheumatoid arthritis. Tapping with the index finger over the carpal tunnel will often bring on paraesthesia (Tinel's sign). Nerve conduction studies will help to confirm the diagnosis.

A wrist splint worn at night or during activity which causes the symptoms may help. If not, depot corticosteroid injection to the carpal tunnel may alleviate symptoms. If the pain is severe, however, and a

Table 8.5 Conditions that predispose to osteomyelitis

Vascular insufficiency, e.g. diabetes mellitus
Soft tissue infection contiguous with bone, e.g. decubitus ulcer
Bacteraemia
Recurrent urinary tract infection
Internal fixation devices

splint and steroid injections have not helped, then surgical retinaculum release under local anaesthetic is the treatment of choice.

8.15 AGE-RELATED MYOPATHIES

8.15.1 Steroid Myopathy

Patients taking high doses of oral corticosteroids over a prolonged period of time may develop a myopathy involving the hip and shoulder musculature. Muscles are weak but not tender and in contrast to inflammatory myositis, muscle enzymes and electromyogram are normal. It should resolve with a reduction in dose and an exercise programme but recovery may take many months.

8.15.2 Osteomalacic Myopathy

Osteomalacia may present with proximal myopathy associated with weakness and wasting. The combination of bone pain and myopathy give rise to a waddling gait. Following treatment with vitamin D the muscle power returns to normal within 3 months.

8.15.3 Hypokalaemic Myopathy

Manifestations of hypokalaemia usually occur at potassium concentrations below 3.5 mmol/l and include muscle weakness, hyporeflexia, paraesthesia, cramps, rhabdomyolysis and paralysis. Symptoms improve with the correction of the underlying hypokalaemia.

FURTHER READING

Akil M, Amos RS. ABC of rheumatology: rheumatoid arthritis. *Br Med J* 1995; 310:587–590, 652–655.

Campbell G, Compston J, Crisp A (eds). *The Management of Common Metabolic Bone Disorders*. Cambridge University Press, Cambridge, 1993.

Gray RG, Gottlieb NL. Intra-articular corticosteroids. An updated assessment. *Clin Orthop* 1983; 177:235–263.

Michet CJ, Evans JM, Fleming KC et al. Common rheumatological disease in elderly patients. *Mayo Clin Proc* 1995; 70:1205–1214.

Millar-Blair DJ, Robbins DL. Rheumatoid arthritis: new science, new treatment. *Geriatrics* 1993; 48:28–38.

Reveille JD. Soft-tissue rheumatism: diagnosis and treatment. *Am J Med* 1997; 102:23S–29S.

Chapter 9

Cancer

9.1 CANCER THERAPY IN OLD AGE: GENERAL CONSIDERATIONS

Most cancer patients are elderly, yet until recent years, such patients have often been excluded from attempts at curative treatment on the grounds that such treatment was considered too rigorous for this age group to tolerate. This view has applied particularly to cytotoxic chemotherapy. In recent years, however, inclusion of elderly patients in large, randomized studies of surgery, radiotherapy and/or chemotherapy for the common cancers has considerably clarified the role of these regimens in treating elderly cancer patients. Age per se should not be a reason for withholding curative therapy. Rather, the prime considerations should be physiological function, estimated life expectancy prior to diagnosis of cancer and patient choice. Therefore, whilst it may be inappropriate to subject many elderly patients to rigorous cancer treatment aimed at cure or significant remission because of poor functional reserve, careful patient selection will usually result in clinical outcomes comparable to those in the general population.

There are a number of **important physiological ageing factors** (see also Chapter 1) in considering elderly patients for cancer therapy. These are listed in Table 9.1. Because of reduced physiological reserve and the higher prevalence of comorbid medical conditions with concurrent drug therapy, careful pretreatment evaluation encompassing general performance, nutrition and social support status are essential in older patients being considered for cancer therapy.

9.2 LUNG CANCER

Although there has been a steady increase in total mortality from lung cancer worldwide over the last 20–25 years, death rates from lung cancer

Table 9.1 Physiological ageing factors that influence cancer therapy

---

(i) Delayed and diminished bone marrow recovery following myelosuppressive chemotherapy.

(ii) Reduced renal blood flow and glomerular filtration leading to reduced renal clearance of some cytotoxics (e.g. methotrexate, cisplatin, bleomycin).

(iii) Reduced liver size, blood flow and oxidative capacity.

(iv) Increased risk of cardiac failure from exposure to potentially cardiotoxic drugs (e.g. doxorubicin) and high-dose chest radiotherapy.

(v) Increased risk of acute confusion from exposure to radiotherapy for malignant glioma, cerebral metastases.

(vi) Slower rate of wound healing and mucous membrane healing following surgery and chemotherapy-induced mucositis respectively.

(vii) Diarrhoea and temporary malabsorption associated with cytotoxic chemotherapy may be more protracted.

---

in the same period in males at all ages in the UK have been declining. The latter trend is due to the fact that men are now smoking less than in previous decades. In contrast, death rates in females over 60 have been climbing steeply, reflecting the ever increasing proportion of women who smoke since the 1940s. Although the number of men with lung cancer currently exceeds the number of women with the disease by a factor of approximately 3, it is anticipated that lung cancer rates in women will match or exceed those in men by the year 2025. The current annual incidence of lung cancer among males aged >65 in the USA is almost 5/1000. Unlike most other common cancers, lung cancer in persons aged over 80 is twice as likely to be localized as lung cancer presenting in middle age, i.e. <50 years. However, the older the patient with lung cancer, the more undifferentiated the tumour is likely to be. This and the cumulative effects of other chronic diseases largely explain why advanced age is linked with poorer survival with lung cancer, i.e. 2-year survival rate of 15% among those under 60, compared to about 5% among those over 70.

Treatment of lung cancer in old age, as with younger age groups, involves surgery, radiotherapy and cytotoxic chemotherapy, and the various combinations of these modalities. Survival after treatment is determined by tumour staging and histological type at diagnosis, and by physiological status. Squamous cell carcinoma is the commonest histological type in elderly people (30%), followed by small cell carcinoma

(24%), adenocarcinoma (22%), large cell carcinoma (22%) and mixed cell carcinoma (2%). Small cell cancers by their nature tend to metastasize early, so that surgery seldom has an important treatment role and chemotherapy is the mainstay of disease-attenuating management. The other critical determinant of treatment option and survival is disease staging. In non-small cell cancers, surgery may be considered for localized disease. However, few elderly patients with lung cancer have enough respiratory reserve to make surgery a realistic option. If the preoperative forced expiratory volume in 1 second (FEV_1) is less than 2 litres, the likelihood of serious post-pneumonectomy respiratory morbidity is greatly increased. However, with FEV_1 values as low as 1.5 litres, lobectomy may be safe provided the surgeon is confident of not having to proceed to full pneumonectomy to achieve a cure. Postoperative mortality with lobectomy in elderly patients is about 3% compared to 15% with pneumonectomy. Operative risk may also be usefully assessed by measuring forced vital capacity (FVC), with risk rising significantly when the age- and gender-adjusted FVC falls below 70% of the predicted value, and rising steeply when FVC is less than 50% of predicted.

Radiotherapy may be curative in some patients with localized tumours and medical contraindications to surgery. Five-year survival rates of approximately 20% may be expected in such patients; however, 5-year survival drops to just 5% with localized tumours of more than 3 cm in diameter. Most elderly patients do not tolerate radical radiotherapy, and the main role of radiotherapy in elderly cases of lung cancer is to palliate symptoms of bleeding, dyspnoea, pain and cough from the primary tumour and local pain from bony metastases.

Cytotoxic chemotherapy is the mainstay of treatment for small cell tumours, and the response rates and toxicity are similar in younger and elderly patient groups. Although 25–30% of patients will achieve early remission, 2-year survival rate is dismal (2–12%), and elderly patients are more likely to experience toxicity, particularly with **carboplatin**, the principal agent in most polychemotherapy regimens. Although carboplatin is better tolerated than cisplatin in terms of nephrotoxicity, neurotoxicity and ototoxicity, carboplatin is more myelosuppressive. Thus, chemotherapy is not a useful option for most elderly patients with small cell lung cancer. However, oral **etoposide** as a single agent has been shown to extend median survival by 9–12 months in limited small cell cancer, and by 8–9.5 months in extensive small cell cancer. Its toxicity is usually low, but unpredictable myelosuppression may occur due to wide variation in bioavailability. However, the survival benefit from etoposide alone is not as good as with polychemotherapy regimens.

Good palliation is the main focus of lung cancer treatment in old age. The main problems specifically associated with lung cancer are dyspnoea, chest pain, haemoptysis, cough and superior vena cava (SVC) obstruction (see Chapter 14). **Dyspnoea** affects 75% of terminally ill lung cancer patients and may have many causes. As well as continuous **humidified oxygen**, patients may get useful symptomatic relief with **morphine/diamorphine**, preferably by continuous subcutaneous infusion. Benzodiazepines may be useful in anxious dyspnoeic patients, e.g. diazepam 2–5 mg three times daily, reducing over several days to a maintenance dose of 2–5 mg nocte. **Dexamethasone** (20 mg immediately, followed by 4–16 mg daily) may reduce **tumour obstruction of the SVC or bronchus**. More recently, endovascular and endobronchial stents have been used with success to relieve large vessel and bronchial obstruction.

9.3 BREAST CANCER

About half of all new cases of breast cancer occur in women aged over 65. Traditionally, many clinicians have regarded breast cancer in older women as a less aggressive disease than in younger women and therefore tended to manage elderly patients conservatively with tamoxifen therapy only. However, current opinion does not support this view and there is a growing body of evidence that the prognosis of elderly women with breast cancer is significantly improved if there is early specialist surgical and oncological referral. The assumption that healthy elderly women do not tolerate or gain as much benefit from surgery, radiotherapy or chemotherapy has no firm basis and at all ages, survival with breast cancer is principally determined by tumour size, nodal status and differentiation. **Stage I** (tumour size <2 cm, no axillary nodal involvement) **and stage II cancer** (axillary nodal involvement and/or tumour >2 cm) is treated by wide local excision or mastectomy plus postoperative radiotherapy plus tamoxifen. Radiotherapy and tamoxifen both reduce the risk of local recurrence (about 30% over 5 years without radiotherapy). Radiotherapy is usually reserved for patients undergoing wide local excision, rather than those having mastectomy.

Tamoxifen (20 mg daily) is both an oestrogen receptor antagonist and partial agonist, and exerts its anti-cancer effect by oestrogen antagonism. It prolongs both disease-free and total survival in elderly women, particularly those with high concentrations of oestrogen and/or progesterone receptors. However, it is also beneficial in some women (about 10%) with a low concentration of tumour cell oestrogen receptors. Tamoxifen is recommended for at least 2 years in stage I and II disease. Known adverse side-effects from tamoxifen include hot flushes, mild nausea, weight gain and disease 'flare' at the start of treatment and its use is associated with a slight, but significant increased risk of endometrial cancer. In general, however, it is well tolerated, even by frail elderly women. In women over 70 in whom there are contra-indications to surgery and radiotherapy, tamoxifen keeps stage I and II breast cancer in remission in about 40% of cases over a 5-year period. Careful follow-up of all women who have had surgery and radiotherapy is indicated, with annual check-ups involving complete physical examination and mammography to detect recurrence or new tumour.

Stage III breast cancer (fixed ipsilateral lymph nodes and/or tumour >5 cm) is associated with a high probability of distant micrometastatic spread and is seldom curable, but may be brought into remission by the combination of partial mastectomy (or radical radiotherapy) and cytotoxic chemotherapy. The cytotoxic agents usually deployed are cyclophosphamide, methotrexate and 5-fluorouracil or doxorubicin and cyclophosphamide. This approach gives a median 5-year survival rate of 40–50%. The survival benefit from tamoxifen in stage III disease is unclear. However, a recent meta-analysis showed that women with breast cancer over the age of 50 treated with tamoxifen alone had similar prolongation of quality-adjusted life and symptom-free survival to those women treated with combined cytotoxic chemotherapy and tamoxifen. Also, recent trials show that the method of local tumour treatment (i.e. conservative surgery, radical mastectomy, radiotherapy) does not influence survival, so that 5-, 10- and 15-year survival rates for each modality are equivalent.

Stage IV disease (distant metastases) is best managed by hormonal therapy, usually **tamoxifen**. In patients with bony metastases, disease suppression is possible with most anti-oestrogen therapies, including tamoxifen and the **aromatase inhibitors** (e.g. aminoglutethimide, anastrozole, formestane and letrozole). Aminoglutethimide achieves good symptom control of advanced cancer, but may not be tolerated by frailer patients. The usual dose in breast cancer is 250 mg once or twice per day. Aminoglutethimide, as an aromatase inhibitor, blocks conversion of adrenal androgens to oestrogens, but also suppresses adrenal glucocorticoid secretion, so that replacement therapy with hydrocortisone is necessary. This is not a requirement with the selective, non-steroidal aromatase inhibitors, anastrozole and letrozole, which may therefore be preferable in older patients in whom drug compliance may be problematic. Tamoxifen causes a tumour flare-up with hypercalcaemia in a minority of patients with bony metastases, which usually settles with intravenous hydration and pamidronate or clodronate, allowing the patient to continue taking tamoxifen. In some patients who are no longer responding to tamoxifen, **progestogens may restabilize metastatic disease**. **Medroxyprogesterone acetate** (400–1500 mg daily) or **megestrol** (160 mg daily in single or divided doses) are suitable progestogenic agents. Their use may be associated with mood swings, abdominal bloating and constipation.

9.4 COLORECTAL CANCER

As with most cancers, elderly people account for the majority of newly presenting cases of colorectal cancer (70–75%). Survival is determined primarily by staging at diagnosis and there is no evidence that colorectal cancer presents at a more advanced stage in elderly patients, who can be expected to have similar survival rates after surgery as younger patients. The mainstay of curative treatment is surgery, since the tumours are only partially radiosensitive and chemosensitive. Patients with Dukes' A cancer have actuarial cancer-free 5-year survival of over 90%. Dukes' B cancer (penetration of the muscularis mucosae, but no evidence of spread to local lymph nodes) carries 50–80% 5-year survival, whilst 5-year survival with Dukes' C cancer (involvement of regional lymph nodes) drops to 30–40%. Patients with Dukes' D cancer (distant metastases) have only a 5–15% likelihood of being alive at 5 years. Patients with Dukes' C colorectal cancer have improved survival rates following adjuvant chemotherapy with 5-fluorouracil combined with folinic acid, which enhances the response rate to 5-fluorouracil.

Many elderly patients do not cope well with a colostomy, so every effort should be made to achieve end-to-end anastomosis from the initial surgery (usually possible except with distal rectal tumours). Even those patients with Dukes' D cancers should be offered surgery if survival is estimated at more than a few months, particularly when there is a high risk of colorectal obstruction or major bleeding, which may be difficult to control by non-surgical means.

9.5 PROSTATE CANCER

Prostate cancer is now the most prevalent cancer in males, accounting for approximately 20% of all newly diagnosed cancers in men. It is also the second most common cause of male cancer mortality. The prevalence of prostate cancer has risen sharply in tandem with increased life expectancy over the last century, and has been described as 'the epidemic in waiting' in view of the increasing proportions of the male population living into old age (age being the strongest risk factor). Prostate cancer accounts for approximately 10 000 deaths in England and Wales every year. However, more prostate cancers are being detected at an earlier stage than previously, due in part to more widespread use of the plasma tumour marker, prostate-specific antigen (PSA) over the last 10 years. Normal PSA levels do not exceed 4 ng/l, but levels rise gradually with age and markedly with prostate cancer, although PSA is not specific for prostate cancer. Levels between 4 and 10 ng/l carry a 20% risk of cancer, whilst levels >10 ng/l have more than a 50% likelihood of cancer, and levels >40 ng/l are consistent with bony metastatic disease. PSA measurement is more sensitive than digital rectal examination (DRE) for detection of early cancers, since cancers are often locally invasive by the time they are detectable by DRE. Over half of all men aged over 70 will have microscopic cancer deposits in the prostate, but only some 2–3% will have symptomatic disease. Diagnosis is confirmed by transrectal ultrasound (TRUS) guided biopsy and disease staging is as follows:

(i)   Stage A: clinically undetectable, discovered incidentally.
(ii) Stage B: tumour palpable, confined to the prostate.
(iii) Stage C: locally invasive disease.
(iv) Stage D: disseminated disease (confirmed by isotope bone scinti-graphy).

The prognosis with prostatic cancer depends on tumour differentiation and whether or not the tumour is confined within the prostate capsule at the time of diagnosis. Poorly differentiated cancers in general carry a 30–60% 10-year mortality rate. However, tumour grade and volume do not appear to influence the rate of cancer progression when the tumour is confined within the prostate. Prostatic cancer may be treated by radical prostatectomy, radical radiotherapy or anti-androgen chemotherapy, depending on the stage of the disease, the health status of the patient and his life expectancy when comorbidity is taken into consideration. In general, patients with localized disease with a life expectancy less than 10 years are not suitable candidates for radical surgery or radiotherapy, since prostate cancer is usually such an indolent disease, usually with a good response to hormonal therapy.

External beam radiotherapy is an attractive treatment option in some elderly patients, where life expectancy is greater than 10 years, and offers equivalent overall survival prospects to radical surgery. Treatment is usually complete by 6–7 weeks and disease-free survival for stage A cancer is 83% and 67% at 5 and 10 years, and 70% and 51% respectively for stage B cancer. Radiotherapy also carries less post-operative morbidity than radical surgery, which can result in persisting incontinence (6–7%), urethral stricture (9–12%) and impotence (30–100%). Rates of these complications are significantly less with radiotherapy. Stage C disease (locally invasive) or pelvic recurrence of stage A and B cancers is palliated with radiotherapy, which can control local disease satisfactorily. Some centres are now treating stage A prostate cancer with **brachytherapy**, i.e. the direct implantation of radioactive seeds under ultrasound or CT guidance using a transrectal or transperi-neal route. These seeds remain in place permanently, giving an intense local dose of radiation. Medium-term results from brachytherapy are at least as good as with optimal surgical management, and brachytherapy has the advantage of being a much less invasive one-day procedure with a lower complication rate compared to surgery.

Localized, asymptomatic disease in elderly men usually requires nothing more than regular surveillance. For metastatic disease, anti-androgen therapy, which offers good symptomatic and survival benefits, is usually indicated. Patients may be offered bilateral subcapsular orchidectomy (under local anaesthesia) or chemical orchidectomy with **luteinizing**

hormone-releasing hormone (LH-RH) agonists. LH-RH agonists cause initial increased LH release from the pituitary, followed by profound LH suppression and secondary hypoandrogenaemia after approximately 1 month. In the first 2–3 weeks of therapy, serum testosterone levels are commonly **increased** as a result of the early LH stimulation. This can cause a tumour 'flare', with transient worsening of metastatic symptoms (e.g. bone pain, spinal cord compression) which may be prevented by premedication with anti-androgens (e.g. **cyproterone acetate** 100 mg two to three times daily or **flutamide** 250 mg three times daily). These work by competing with dihydrotestosterone at receptor level (androgenic effects of testosterone are mediated by conversion to dihydrotestosterone). **Buserelin**, **goserelin**, **leuprorelin** and **triptorelin** are all suitable LH-RH agonists for treating metastatic prostate cancer. Three-monthly subcutaneous injection therapy is also available (e.g. goserelin 10.8 mg) and is convenient for patient and physician. However, since neither orchidectomy nor LH-RH agonists suppress adrenal androgen production, there is a case for concomitant therapy with an anti-androgen. There is some evidence for better symptom control and survival with combined LH-RH agonist and anti-androgen therapy. However, long-term therapy with anti-androgens carries a small risk of serious hepatotoxicity and should be stopped when there is evidence of deranged liver enzymes.

Cytotoxic chemotherapy for palliation of metastatic prostate cancer is generally disappointing, with no more than 10% of patients receiving significantly improved survival (of a few months). External beam radiotherapy offers useful palliation for painful bony metastases.

9.6 GYNAECOLOGICAL CANCERS

Endometrial, cervical and ovarian tumours account for more than 90% of cases of gynaecological malignancy. These tumours tend to present at a more advanced stage in elderly women than in younger women, and therefore have a worse prognosis in old age. Nevertheless, elderly women given the same treatment at the same disease stage as younger women have similar survival rates.

Endometrial cancer is the most common gynaecological malignancy. Fortunately, it usually presents with **stage I or II disease** (i.e. confined to the uterus), and is therefore **usually curable by total abdominal hysterectomy and bilateral salpingo-oophorectomy** (TAH/BSO). **Stage III** (pelvic lymph node or peritoneal involvement) **and stage IV** (spread to adjacent viscera or liver) **disease is usually managed by radiotherapy, progestogens (e.g. megestrol acetate 40 mg four times daily) and/or chemotherapy**. As many as 40% of patients with metastatic disease will have an objective response to progestogen therapy alone, and survival is significantly improved in these patients. Combination chemotherapy (e.g. cyclophosphamide, doxorubicin and cisplatin; CAP) increases the objective response rate, but is seldom appropriate for elderly patients because of its toxicity.

Cervical cancer is curable with surgery or radiotherapy in 80–90% of women with stage I disease. More advanced disease is usually treated with radiotherapy alone, although some bulky tumours are resected wholly or partially prior to irradiation. The overall cure rate for cervical cancer is 50–60%. Cervical cancer is not particularly chemosensitive.

Ovarian cancers, in contrast, are among the most chemosensitive of all tumours. Management is usually by **TAH/BSO for stage I or II disease**. **Carboplatin** as a single agent is the primary treatment for **stage III and IV disease, following prior tumour debulking surgery**. The dose of carboplatin is adjusted according to renal function because it is potentially nephrotoxic. Few surgeons perform a 'second-look' laparotomy in elderly patients to estimate long-term prognosis more accurately following primary debunking surgery and adjuvant combination chemotherapy (as used in younger women) because of increased postoperative morbidity and mortality following further major surgery.

9.7 LYMPHOMA

Hodgkin's disease (HD) shows a bimodal age distribution, with the second peak occurring between age 60 and 65 years. Non-Hodgkin's lymphoma (NHL) similarly is not uncommon in elderly people, about 30% of cases occurring in the over-70s. Lymphoma tends to present at more advanced disease stages in the elderly compared to young people and the intensive radiotherapy and chemotherapy regimens used are less well tolerated, so that lower doses are used. For these reasons, lymphoma carries a poorer prognosis in this age group. Despite this, HD is still a curable disease in most elderly patients with stage I and II disease, and 30–40% of patients with stage III and IV disease achieve long-term survival with treatment. Table 9.2 gives details of the staging of HD. **Adverse prognostic factors in HD** include:

- bulk disease (i.e. massive adenopathy)
- 'B' symptoms (i.e. fever, night sweats, weight loss)
- age >60
- elevated plasma lactate dehydrogenase (LDH)
- mixed cellularity or lymphocyte depleted histology
- involvement of more than three nodal sites.

In general, radiotherapy is the recommended treatment for stage I and II disease, and chemotherapy ± radiotherapy for stage III and IV disease. The two most widely used chemotherapy regimens for HD are ChlVPP and derivations of ABVD. ChlVPP comprises **chl**orambucil, **v**inblastine, **p**rednisolone and **p**rocarbazine. The ABVD protocol includes **a**driamycin (doxorubicin), **b**leomycin, **v**inblastine and **d**acarbazine. Chemotherapy cycles are repeated every 4 weeks for 6–12 cycles and two cycles beyond complete remission, but doses may need to be reduced by half to two-thirds in elderly patients to avoid treatment intolerance.

Non-Hodgkin's lymphoma is staged in a similar manner to HD. In addition, NHL is graded as low-, intermediate- and high-grade on the basis of tumour histology. Treatment (radiotherapy and combination chemotherapy) is given on the basis of tumour staging and grading. **Elderly patients with stage I or II nodular disease without symptoms (low-grade NHL) usually do not require treatment**. When symptoms

Table 9.2   Staging of Hodgkin's lymphoma

Stage	Description
I	Disease limited to one lymph node region
II	2 or more lymph node regions involved on same side of diaphragm
III	Lymph node involvement on both sides of diaphragm (spleen, tonsils, adenoids considered as lymph nodes)
IV	Disseminated involvement of 1 or more extranodal areas (e.g. bone marrow, liver) ± lymph node involvement

arise, local irradiation can be used alone or in combination with chemotherapy. With intermediate- and high-grade (diffuse, symptomatic) disease or stage III/IV disease, chemotherapy is usually indicated, but the combination regimens used in younger patients (e.g. CHOP—cyclophosphamide, doxorubicin, vincristine (Oncovin) and prednisolone) tend to be less well tolerated in elderly patients. For this reason, other less toxic regimens such as 'mini-CHOP' (CHOP with lower dose doxorubicin) or CNOP (CHOP with mitozantrone instead of doxorubicin) are used.

9.8   SKIN CANCERS

The major skin cancers in old age are basal cell carcinoma (BCC), squamous cell carcinoma (SCC) and malignant melanoma. **Basal cell carcinoma** usually presents on the head and neck, has a nodular, pearly appearance and sometimes ulcerates in the centre as it expands ('rodent ulcer'). Although BCCs seldom metastasize, they may invade local tissues, causing destruction of bone, muscle and cartilage with resultant disfiguration and pain. Biopsy-proven BCCs are usually treated by **simple surgical excision, curettage or cryotherapy**. Large or recurrent BCCs may be treated by surgical excision. **Radiotherapy** is useful for BCCs that present problems for surgical excision (e.g. eyelid tumours) and for better cosmetic results. Topical 5-fluorouracil is generally not recommended for BCC, in view of the high recurrence rate on stopping treatment.

Squamous cell carcinoma, unlike BCCs, may metastasize and therefore requires ablation without delay. **Simple surgical excision**, **cryotherapy** and **radiotherapy** are the usual treatment options. Excision is recommended for single, small, well-differentiated SCCs, cryotherapy for multiple SCCs and radiotherapy for poorly differentiated and recurrent tumours. Premalignant lesions (usually actinic keratoses) should be removed.

The incidence of **malignant melanoma** has approximately trebled in the last 40 years. This is thought to relate to ever increasing levels of sun exposure in the at-risk white population. Most cases occur in elderly people, and the following clinical features in a pigmented naevus should raise suspicion:

- asymmetry
- border irregularity
- colour variegation
- diameter >6 mm
- elevation from the skin surface.

The depth of tumour cell infiltration (the Breslow level) is the prime determinant of prognosis, since melanoma is poorly chemosensitive and radiosensitive. Patients with tumour invasion to a depth of less than 1 mm have a 5-year disease-free survival of over 90%, whilst a tumour thickness >3.65 mm carries a high risk of metastatic disease (i.e. 60–70% over 8 years' follow-up). Therefore, clinical follow-up every 6–12 months is mandatory for patients with tumours that penetrate to a depth of >1.70 mm. Lentigo maligna of the face, head or neck is the most common form of melanoma in the over-65s, in contrast to superficial spreading melanoma in younger people. It is a slowly expanding brown or black lesion, often on the cheek, that commonly develops into a nodule (invasive lentigo maligna melanoma). Melanoma often presents

Table 9.3 The Glasgow 7-Point Checklist for suspected melanoma

Malignant transformation in a new, pre-existent or pigmented lesion is suggested by the following:

(A) 3 major points:
- change in shape
- change in size
- change in colour

(B) 4 minor points:
- oozing or bleeding
- size >6 mm
- inflammation
- itching

Key:
1 or more major points: refer for dermatological assessment
1 major point and 1 or more minor points: excision biopsy
4 minor points: refer for dermatological assessment

Adapted from: MacKie R. Melanoma. Presentation and treatment in the elderly. *Geriatr Med* 1997; 27:31–36.

at an advanced, locally invasive stage in elderly people, possibly because lesions are dismissed by patients and doctors as non-specific, age-related benign lesions. When assessing pigmented lesions, the Glasgow 7-Point Checklist (Table 9.3) is helpful for deciding who should be referred for specialist dermatological assessment. **Excision biopsy with a margin of 1 cm of normal skin** is the procedure of choice, and can usually be done under local anaesthesia.

9.9   ONCOLOGICAL EMERGENCIES

The common emergencies in cancer patients are infection, vertebral collapse with spinal cord compression, pathological fracture, acute

Table 9.4   Management of common oncological emergencies

Condition	Investigation	Treatment
(1) Infection	Specimen culture Leucocyte count	Intravenous antibiotics; relieve associated obstruction (e.g. bronchial, biliary)
(2) Spinal cord compression	Plain X-rays of spine CT/MRI scan of spine	Radiotherapy or surgical decompression (e.g. bronchial, colorectal, renal cell metastases)
(3) Pathological fracture	Plain X-rays ± isotope scintigraphy	Orthopaedic internal fixation ± prophylactic radiotherapy to other at-risk lesions
(4) Hypercalcaemia	U&E Alkaline phosphatase Plain X-rays Isotope scintigraphy	Rehydration and diuresis (intravenous saline ± frusemide) Bisphosphonate infusion
(5) Hyponatraemia	U&E Plasma and urine osmolarity (SIADH) Short synacthen test	Restrict fluid if SIADH Intravenous saline if dehydrated Hydrocortisone if hypoadrenalism
(6) Hyperuricaemia	Plasma urate, U&E, urinary urate, U&E	Hydration, allopurinol
(7) Vena caval obstruction	Cavography	Radiotherapy ± caval stent insertion

CT/MRI, computed tomography/magnetic resonance imaging; U&E, urea and electrolytes; SIADH, syndrome of inappropriate antidiuretic hormone secretion.

metabolic disorder (e.g. hypercalcaemia, hyponatraemia, hyperuricaemic renal failure) and vena caval obstruction. Table 9.4 details the management of these problems.

The management of haematological malignancies is discussed in Chapter 12. Palliation of common problems in terminal cancer is discussed in Chapter 14.

FURTHER READING

Gelber RD, Cole BF, Goldhirsch A et al. Adjuvant chemotherapy plus tamoxifen compared to tamoxifen for postmenopausal breast cancer: meta-analysis of quality-adjusted survival. *Lancet* 1996; 347:1066–1071.

Kirby RS, Christmas TJ, Brawen M. *Prostate Cancer.* Mosby, London, 1996.

Lichtman SM, Bayer RL. Gastrointestinal cancer in the elderly. *Clin Geriatr Med* 1997; 13:307–326.

McKenna RJ Sr. Clinical aspects of cancer in the elderly: treatment decisions, treatment choices and follow-up. *Cancer* 1994; 74:2107–2117.

Vose JM. Non-Hodgkin's lymphoma. In: RE Rakel (ed). *Conn's Current Therapy.* WB Saunders Company, Philadelphia, 1995, pp 374–377.

Williams C. Adjuvant systemic therapies for breast cancer. *Prescriber J* 1996; 36:125–129.

Chapter 10

Urogenital Disorders

10.1 URINARY TRACT INFECTION

Urinary tract infections (UTIs) are common in elderly people, with an annual incidence of 5–10%. This relatively high incidence is related to several factors. In females, genital atrophy due to reduced oestrogen results in loss of the relatively acidic pH of the vagina, allowing colonization with potentially pathogenic faecal flora. In males, the increased prevalence of bladder outflow obstruction due to benign prostatic hyperplasia associated with post-voiding residual urine increases the risk of infection. In both sexes, constipation with faecal impaction, faecal soiling of the perineum and indwelling bladder catheters predispose to UTI. The treatment of UTI depends on a number of factors other than the particular pathogen identified. These include:

- the presence or absence of symptoms
- localization (i.e. whether there is cystitis or pyelonephritis)
- whether infection is recurrent or sporadic, and
- whether the UTI is complicated or not.

The patient's gender is also relevant when interpreting urine microscopy/culture reports, since the threshold for significant bacteriuria in females is $>10^2$ colony-forming units/ml of urine, whilst in males it is $>10^5$ colony-forming units/ml. For bacteriuria to be clinically significant, i.e. to warrant antibiotic treatment, the patient must be symptomatic and there must be pyuria on microscopy, i.e. >10 leucocytes/µl of urine. Asymptomatic bacteriuria is common, particularly among those with post-void residual urine and bladder catheters, but should not lead to attempts to sterilize the urine with antibiotics, since relapse is highly likely and antibiotic resistance is promoted. Also, there is no firm evidence that treatment prevents symptomatic UTI.

The pathogens associated with UTI in older people differ somewhat from those seen in younger people (Table 10.1), with a smaller proportion due to *Escherichia coli* than in younger people, i.e. 60–70% versus 80–90%. In elderly women with community-acquired UTI, the pathogen isolate distribution is approximately as follows: *E. coli* 60–70%, non-*E. coli* Gram-negative organisms (*Proteus, Klebsiella, Pseudomonas*) 15–20% and Gram-positive organisms (mostly *Staphylococcus* and *Enterococcus* species) 15–20%. In elderly men, Gram-positive organisms account for 30–40% of isolates. Confirmation of a significant UTI may be difficult, particularly in frail elderly people. This may be due to factors such as non-specific symptoms (e.g. malaise, confusion, anorexia) and inability to obtain a 'clean-catch' mid-stream specimen of urine. In these circumstances, particularly in females, a representative urine sample may be obtained by passing a bladder catheter, which is removed immediately the sample is obtained. Alternatively, in males and females, an uncontaminated urine sample may be obtained by puncture aspiration of a full bladder under aseptic technique. However, for safety one must confirm a full bladder (e.g. using portable ultrasound equipment). Immediate dipstick analysis for blood, protein, nitrite and leucocyte esterase is helpful for rapid diagnosis, since the presence of nitrite and leucocyte esterase makes UTI highly likely and empiric therapy may be started immediately. If urgent treatment is required in a very ill patient, urine samples should be immediately analysed by microscopy for leucocytes, Gram-negative or Gram-positive organisms as well as the presence of cellular casts, indicating pyelonephritis. Until the pathogen is identified and its antibiotic sensitivities confirmed, suitable empiric therapy for community-acquired infections is **trimethoprim** 200 mg twice daily for uncomplicated cystitis and **ciprofloxacin** 200 mg twice daily intravenously for pyelonephritis (Table 10.1).

With **hospital-acquired or nursing-home-acquired UTIs**, *E. coli*, *Proteus, Pseudomonas, Enterococcus, Klebsiella, Morganella* and *Providentia* are commonly isolated. **Trimethoprim** is the usual empiric first-line therapy for nosocomial cystitis. Second-line therapy with broader-spectrum agents (e.g. **fluoroquinolones**) is indicated if patients fail to improve after 48 hours' therapy with trimethoprim or urine culture results confirm trimethoprim resistance. Similarly, a higher incidence of resistant organisms in cases of pyelonephritis means that **intravenous broad-spectrum drugs** such as fluoroquinolones (e.g.

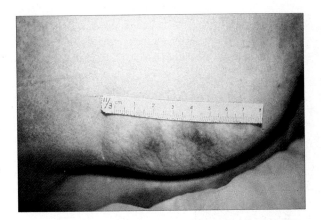

Plate I Grade 1 pressure sore on buttocks

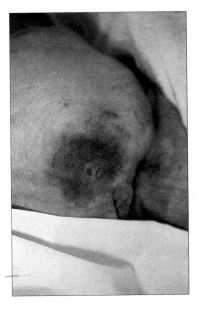

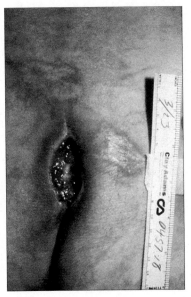

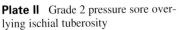

Plate II Grade 2 pressure sore over-lying ischial tuberosity

Plate III Grade 3 pressure sore over sacrum

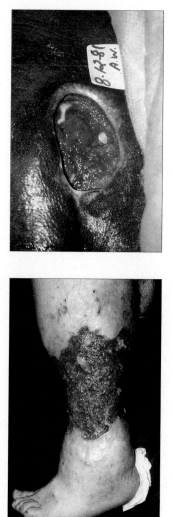

Plate IV Grade 4 pressure sore over sacrum (Plates I–IV courtesy of Mrs C. Dealey)

Plate V Circumferential mixed arterial and venous leg ulceration with secondary lymphoedema

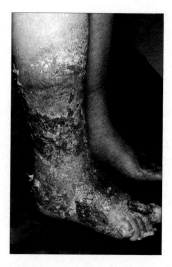

Plate VI Venous leg ulceration with secondarily infected allergic contact dermatitis due to rubber in compression bandages (note also severe onychogryphosis)

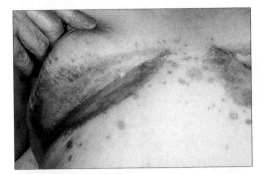

Plate VII
Submammary candidal intertrigo

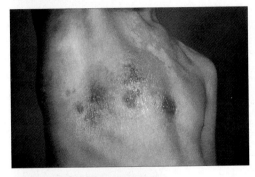

Plate VIII
Herpes zoster rash affecting right fifth thoracic dermatome (note typical vesicular appearance)

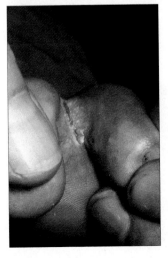

Plate IX
Tinea pedis with interdigital maceration

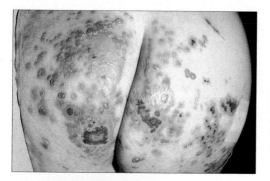

Plate X
Bullous pemphigoid eruption (note tense blisters on a background urticarial eruption)

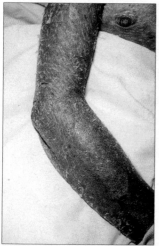

Plate XI
Erythroderma (generalized eruption)

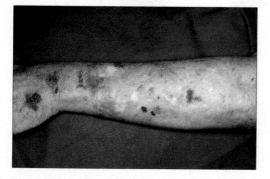

Plate XII
Corticosteroid purpura accentuated by age-related dermal atrophy (Plates V–XII courtesy of Dr G. Stewart)

Table 10.1 Treatment of urinary tract infection*

Classification	Empiric antibiotic choice and dosage	Treatment duration	Pathogens
Community-acquired cystitis	1st: trimethoprim 200 mg b.i.d. 2nd: cephalexin 250 mg q.i.d.	5 days	E. coli
Relapsed cystitis	Same antibiotic if sensitive		
Community-acquired pyelonephritis	1st: ciprofloxacin 200 mg b.i.d. IV 2nd: cefuroxime 750 mg t.i.d. IV (switch to oral therapy when symptoms settled >24 h)	14 days	E. coli Proteus Klebsiella Enterococci Staphylococci
Hospital-acquired cystitis	1st: trimethoprim 200 mg b.i.d. 2nd: ciprofloxacin 250 mg b.i.d.	5 days	E. coli Proteus Klebsiella Pseudomonas Providentia Morganella
Hospital-acquired pyelonephritis	1st: ciprofloxacin 200–400 mg b.i.d. IV 2nd: cefotaxime or ceftazidime 1 g t.i.d. IV	14 days	E. coli Proteus Klebsiella Pseudomonas Providentia Morganella
Acute prostatitis	1st: ciprofloxacin 250 mg b.i.d. 2nd: amoxycillin 500 mg q.i.d. plus gentamicin 1–1.5 mg/kg b.i.d.	4 weeks (at least)	E. coli Proteus Klebsiella Pseudomonas Enterococci
Recurrent UTI prophylaxis	1st: trimethoprim 50–100 mg nocte 2nd: nitrofurantoin 50–100 mg nocte	Continuous	Proteus Klebsiella Pseudomonas Enterococci

*Urinary tract infection is defined as being symptomatic and confirmed by finding $>10^2$ colony-forming units (CFUs) in females or 10^5 CFUs in males with >10 leucocytes/μl of urine.

b.i.d., twice daily; t.i.d., three times daily; q.i.d., four times daily.

ciprofloxacin 200 mg twice daily or **ofloxacin** 200 mg once daily) or third-generation cephalosporins (e.g. **cefotaxime** 1 g three times daily or **ceftazidime** 1 g three times daily) are recommended for seriously ill patients. **Ampicillin or amoxycillin is not recommended** as first-line therapy for community-acquired infections, because of the high rate of *E. coli* resistance (13–30%), although there is less resistance with beta-lactamase stable coamoxiclav. Cystitis should be treated for 5 days and pyelonephritis for 14 days. With pyelonephritis, intravenous therapy should be maintained until the patient's pyrexia has abated, following which oral antibiotics are appropriate. The choice of oral antibiotic should be on the basis of reported sensitivities with urine culture.

Prolonged antibiotic therapy is also required in so-called '**complicated UTI**'. These include cases with associated urinary tact obstruction, incomplete bladder emptying (e.g. urethral stricture, neurogenic bladder) and a persistent focus of infection such as prostatitis, chronic indwelling bladder catheter or renal abscess. The most common causes of compli-cated UTI are bladder outflow obstruction and in-dwelling bladder catheter. All patients having long-term bladder catheterization develop bacteriuria, usually within 10–14 days, even with closed drainage systems. **Antibiotic therapy for asymptomatic bacteriuria in cathe-terized patients is not recommended**. Symptomatic infection risk is minimized by maintaining a high fluid intake and attention to hygiene. Cell debris commonly lodges in the inner lining of the catheter and acts as a focus for bacterial colonization and infection. **Catheter obstruction** may result from debris build-up and should be managed by changing the catheter. Bladder irrigation to clear obstruc-tion is not recommended since it may result in bacterial reflux into the ureters and kidneys with resultant infection and bacteraemia. Regular changing of bladder catheters is no longer recommended, provided there is free drainage of urine and the patient is asymptomatic. **Catheter-associated UTIs** should be treated in the same way as in patients without catheters (see Table 10.1). However, it should be appreciated that the organism(s) identified from culture of catheter-derived urine specimens may not be the organism causing the cystitis or pyelo-nephritis, since a variety of organisms may colonize the lining of the catheter. Therefore blood cultures and culture of the first urine sample taken after insertion of a new bladder catheter (or from bladder puncture) are helpful in identifying the pathogen.

Acute prostatitis is not common, but is important to diagnose because antibiotic therapy needs to be prolonged over several weeks. Typical symptoms of acute dysuria or urinary obstruction, pyrexia, perineal or low back pain should arouse suspicion, and the prostate is usually tender on rectal palpation. Prostatic massage is useful to obtain prostatic fluid for culture, but may cause bacteraemia, and should be followed immediately with intravenous antibiotics. The drugs of choice are fluoroquinolones, such as **ciprofloxacin** 250 mg twice daily or **ofloxacin** 200–400 mg daily. Analgesia, hydration and stool softeners are also important for symptom relief. Antibiotic therapy should be continued for 4 weeks and the patient carefully reassessed with repeat urine culture 1 month after stopping antibiotics. **Chronic prostatitis** may be the cause of persistent bacteriuria or recurrent UTI in some men, and may require long-term (i.e. 4–12 weeks) antibiotic therapy with low-dose trimethoprim, nitrofurantoin or a fluoroquinolone, depending on the antibiotic sensitivity.

Prophylactic antibiotics for recurrent UTIs may be necessary in some patients, usually those with urinary tract structural abnormalities that are not surgically correctable. Recommended prophylactic antibiotics include **trimethoprim** 50–100 mg or **nitrofurantoin** 50–100 mg nocte. Nitrofurantoin is not suitable in patients with renal impairment, since bactericidal concentrations in urine are unlikely to be reached and the risk of polyneuropathy (often progressive and irreversible) is increased. Prophylactic therapy is not advised in patients with long-term bladder catheters, since the likelihood of colonization and infection with antibiotic-resistant catheter strains is high. Also, patients undergoing urinary tract instrumentation (e.g. cystoscopy, prostatectomy) who are at risk of endocarditis require prophylaxis beginning 24 hours before the procedure (see Chapter 2). **Intravaginal topical oestrogens** also help prevent recurrent UTIs in older women.

Avoidance of bladder catheters and **regular intake of cranberry juice** (which is thought to reduce the adhesion of bacteria to urothelium) help reduce the incidence of UTIs in elderly people living in long-term care facilities.

10.2   URINARY INCONTINENCE AND BLADDER OUTFLOW OBSTRUCTION

An estimated 12% of elderly women in the community and approximately half of all elderly people living in institutional care settings suffer from urinary incontinence. In addition, elderly men living at home have a 7% prevalence rate of urinary incontinence, emphasizing the fact that urinary incontinence is a very large public health problem indeed. Despite this, urinary incontinence is curable in a significant proportion of elderly people, and if not curable is treatable in all but a few, so that the aim of management should be a complete avoidance of wet clothing and secondary skin problems in all patients.

There are several types of urinary incontinence, each with distinct causes and treatments. Clinical assessment aims to identify the cause(s) of incontinence to form the basis of a logical management plan. Although age-related disorders predispose to incontinence (e.g. genital atrophy in females, prostatic obstruction in males, increased incidence of uninhibited detrusor contractions, increased post-voiding residual urine volume, a tendency to nocturia, diuretic drugs, etc.), ageing per se does not **cause** incontinence. Similarly, disorders of the urogenital tract are not always the cause of urinary incontinence. With so-called '**functional incontinence**', patients have normally functioning bladders but become incontinent because of various problems that restrict their ability to get to a toilet quickly enough, e.g. combination of loop diuretics with concomitant severe arthritis making access to an upstairs toilet difficult. In this instance, treatment to improve the arthritis and better access to an alternative toilet facility such as a nearby commode or a downstairs toilet is likely to cure the incontinence.

Urinary incontinence is usefully classified as **transient** or **established** incontinence, since the aetiologies and prognoses are generally different. **Transient incontinence** occurs in the context of some other medical problem and usually clears up when the underlying problem is resolved (Table 10.2). Transient incontinence may also be caused by **drugs with anticholinergic effects** that impair detrusor contractility leading to urine overflow (e.g. tricyclic antidepressants, low potency neuroleptics), by **sedative drugs** leading to confusion, by **opioid analgesics** that cause constipation and faecal impaction with resultant bladder neck

Table 10.2 Causes and mechanisms of transient incontinence

Cause	Mechanism	Treatment
Acute confusion	Disorientation, disinhibition	Regular toileting, temporary catheter if unsuccessful
Acute immobility	Functional, cannot reach toilet in time	Commode or urine bottle, mobilizing physiotherapy
Acute UTI	Detrusor instability	Antibiotics, regular toileting
Polyuria	Drugs, osmotic diuresis (e.g. diabetes mellitus)	Stop causative drugs, treat underlying metabolic disorder
Faecal impaction	Bladder neck obstruction→overflow incontinence	Temporary catheter, disimpact rectum
Drugs:		
(i) Anticholinergics	Impaired detrusor contractility→overflow incontinence	Stop offending drug
(ii) Sedatives	Confusion→functional incontinence	
(iii) Opioid analgesics	Constipation→faecal impaction	
(iv) Calcium antagonists	Bladder outflow obstruction→overflow incontinence	
(v) Alpha-1 antagonists	Excessive urethral sphincter relaxation→stress incontinence	

obstruction and urine overflow and by **diuretics** causing polyuria. Bladder residual urine volume may be increased by **calcium antagonists**, leading to overflow incontinence. **Alpha-adrenergic agonists** (e.g. phenylpropanolamine and phenylephrine used as nasal decongestants, often sold over the counter) may increase smooth muscle contraction in the bladder neck, which, coupled with bladder outflow obstruction due to prostatic enlargement in men, may lead to urinary retention with overflow incontinence. **Alpha-1-adrenergic antagonists** such as prazosin, terazosin and alfuzosin, which are used to treat incontinence associated with bladder outflow obstruction, may sometimes worsen incontinence by causing excessive smooth muscle relaxation in the bladder neck. Also, **ethanol** with its sedative and diuretic effects can cause incontinence.

Established incontinence may be caused by detrusor overactivity or underactivity or by bladder outlet obstruction or incompetence. Diagnosis may be established in most patients by history, examination and, in some patients, estimation of post-void residual urine volume by portable bladder ultrasound equipment. Table 10.3 summarizes the features of the major types of established incontinence. In addition to the typical symptoms, examination may be revealing, e.g. uterovaginal prolapse, cystocele, rectocele, palpable bladder, atrophic urethritis or vaginitis, pelvic mass, faecal impaction, prostatic tumour, central nervous system signs, peripheral neuropathy, loss of sacral dermatomal sensation or reflexes, dribbling low-flow urinary stream and urinalysis indicating haematuria, glycosuria, proteinuria or nitrite with leucocyte reductase. Post-void residual urine volume may be measured simply by 'in–out' catheterization or portable suprapubic bladder ultrasound scanning (more 'patient-friendly') so that insufficient bladder emptying may be quantified. Urine culture should be sought in all cases, since simple antibiotic therapy may cure some cases of established incontinence with chronic UTI. Further investigation of the urinary tract with cystometry, radiology and cystoscopy are indicated in a minority of selected cases only.

The specific type of incontinence requires a specific management approach, which may be surgical, pharmacological, a combination of these, or palliative. Urinary tract infection and constipation/faecal impaction must be treated with appropriate antibiotics or laxatives. For **stress incontinence**, conservative measures beginning with **pelvic muscle exercises** should be attempted in all patients, even when it is apparent that surgery offers the best prospect of improvement since perioperative morbidity/mortality may be avoidable. Pelvic exercises are not difficult, even in frail elderly women, provided the patient can understand the basic principles and activities involved and receives encouragement and supervision from a trained nurse or physiotherapist. The patient is encouraged to maintain a maximal pelvic contraction for 3–10 seconds and to repeat this exercise 10 times 3–5 times daily, 3–4 days per week. Pelvic exercises may be enhanced in some well-

Table 10.3 Clinical features of established urinary incontinence

Type of incontinence	Typical features	Common causes
(A) Women		
Genuine stress incontinence	Urinary leakage with exertion, raised intra-abdominal pressure (e.g. on voluntary cough)	Pelvic floor incompetence due to obstetric injury, pelvic surgery, postmenopausal atrophy, chronic cough
Mixed stress incontinence/detrusor instability	Combined stress and urgency symptoms	Combined pathology
Bladder fistula	Continuous urinary leakage without retention	Pelvic surgery, radiotherapy Obstetric injury Gynaecological cancer
(B) Men		
Bladder obstruction with overflow	Poor stream, straining, continuous urinary leakage	Prostatic hypertrophy Prostatic cancer Urethral stricture Faecal impaction Pelvic surgery
(C) Both sexes		
Detrusor instability	Urinary frequency, urgency, bladder 'hyperreflexia'	Prostatic hypertrophy Prostatic cancer Bulbourethral stricture Stroke Alzheimer's disease Parkinson's disease Spinal cord lesions Cystitis Idiopathic
Detrusor insufficiency	Poor stream, leakage, straining to void, urinary frequency, loss of awareness of bladder, bladder atonia, high post-void residual volume, overflow incontinence	Uterine, bladder prolapse Neuropathic bladder Pelvic surgery, radiotherapy Pelvic masses

motivated elderly women by use of weighted vaginal cones, i.e. metal cones of ascending weight retained within the vagina whilst in the standing posture for increasing intervals, which helps improve pelvic muscle strength and tone. However, pelvic exercises need to be maintained indefinitely for continuing benefit. **Topical vaginal oestrogen** (e.g. dienoestrol 0.01% cream once daily) or **cyclical oral oestrogens** may also help stress incontinence in some elderly women. Phenylpropanolamine, an alpha-adrenergic agonist, which may promote continence in some younger women, is generally not effective or well-tolerated in elderly women. If conservative measures fail, those who are likely to tolerate surgery should be referred for **pelvic repair**, as this offers the best hope of curing stress incontinence.

With incontinence due to **detrusor instability**, the first line of management is **bladder training**. This involves calculating the average interval between successive bladder voids. The patient is then asked to hold his/her urine for 30 minutes longer before voiding. The urine holding time is gradually increased until, if successful, the patient is able to go for up to 6 hours without the need to void. Other regimens involve encouraging the patient to postpone voiding until a set time point is reached, e.g. voiding by the clock. Alternatively, routine toileting may be based on signs of impending voiding (e.g. restlessness) and checking incontinence pads to estimate the time between successive voids. In the nursing home setting, motivated staff may be able to use knowledge of individual patients' patterns to prevent incontinence by anticipatory toileting. **Anticholinergic drugs** may be helpful, since detrusor contractions are mediated by the parasympathetic innervation of the bladder. **Oxybutinin** (2.5–5 mg three times daily) is a suitable choice for most patients. Alternatives are propantheline, flavoxate and imipramine, but are no more effective than oxybutinin. Anticholinergic drugs may cause serious side-effects in elderly patients, including:

- confusion
- constipation
- urinary retention
- glaucoma
- blurred vision
- dry mouth.

Desmopressin nasal spray (20–40 µg once daily), a synthetic analogue of vasopressin, may be useful as an adjunct to anticholinergic therapy. It works by reducing urine volume and may be particularly helpful for nocturnal incontinence. It is also available in tablet form (200–400 µg nocte), which may be more suitable for frail patients. Fluid intake needs to be restricted whilst the drug is active because of the risk of water retention, volume overload and hyponatraemia. For these reasons, it should be avoided in patients with cardiac failure who may have borderline or definite hyponatraemia from taking loop diuretics, and it is advisable to monitor plasma sodium whilst patients are taking desmopressin. Surgery is seldom helpful for primary detrusor instability.

So-called **bladder hyperreflexia** is another common cause of incontinence associated with neurological disorders. Tonic inhibition of detrusor contraction at cerebral level, which is fundamental to maintaining continence, may be impaired as a result of disorders of CNS function. This results in powerful reflex detrusor contractions when bladder filling reaches the reflex threshold, which is far below bladder capacity. Such patients may also be helped by **oxybutinin**. However, if bladder emptying is incomplete, there is a risk of urinary retention and overflow incontinence with anticholinergic therapy. Therefore, post-void residual volume should always be measured in patients with neurological disorders before starting anticholinergic drugs. Patients with high post-void residual volumes require long-term catheter drainage, unless intermittent catheter drainage is an option (seldom a practical solution in elderly patients). External sphincter weakness may sometimes cause stress incontinence in neurologically impaired patients, which may be compounded by detrusor instability. Occasionally, well selected patients with this problem regain continence with surgical artificial sphincter implantation.

Incontinence due to **bladder outflow obstruction** in men usually occurs with more severe prostatic obstruction, and restoration of urinary flow requires prostatic resection. However, in milder cases, alpha-adrenergic blockers may be helpful. These drugs cause bladder neck relaxation and facilitate bladder emptying. Examples include **prazosin** (0.5–2 mg twice daily), **doxazosin** (2–4 mg daily), **terazosin** (5–10 mg daily) **and alfuzosin** (2.5–5 mg twice daily). None of these drugs selectively block bladder alpha-1-adrenoceptors and they may cause hypotension and dizziness in susceptible patients. They should therefore be used with great caution and careful monitoring for orthostatic hypotension. 5-Alpha-reductase inhibitors (e.g. finasteride) are of doubtful value in more severe prostatism, may take several months to show an effect, carry a risk of masking markers of prostate cancer and are expensive. They are, therefore, not recommended in elderly men. **Secondary detrusor instability** may be a problem with chronic bladder outflow obstruction but may be difficult to detect without urodynamic evaluation. In such cases, a trial of bladder training or oxybutinin may be worthwhile. Similarly, chronic obstruction may lead to an atonic bladder so that even after prostatic resection, the patient continues to have continuous dribbling of urine or overflow incontinence. Such cases (mostly men) usually require long-term condom catheter drainage. Incontinence **following previous prostatic surgery** is usually due to chronic urinary retention with overflow incontinence and may result from urethral stricture, recurrent prostate enlargement or inadequate prostate resection. In these circumstances, patients may need urological referral for stricture dilatation, urethrotomy or revised prostate resection.

Palliation of incontinence with sheath urinals, absorbent pads, occlusive pants (although these may be hot and uncomfortable) and other non-invasive devices should not be underestimated, and may be used as an adjuvant to other therapies if complete continence is not achievable, particularly at night. Close attention must be paid to avoid buttock, sacral and perineal skin damage from contact with urine. Hydrophobic barrier creams (e.g. **dimethicone**) are helpful in this regard. Indwelling bladder catheters (transurethral or suprapubic) should be used only as a last resort for chronic incontinence and should be silicone or silicone-coated, rather than latex. Smaller inflation balloons (i.e. 10 ml) should be used as routine to avoid trauma to the bladder base. Suprapubic catheters may be useful where the urethra cannot be negotiated and the obstruction cannot be removed. They also have the advantage of being easier to change than transurethral catheters in males. Not infrequently, patients are still wet despite bladder catheterization due to urine bypassing the catheter. This is usually due to catheter blockage or detrusor instability. The latter problem may be helped by replacement with a smaller calibre catheter with a smaller capacity balloon. Persistent bypassing despite a change of catheter may sometimes respond to oxybutinin.

10.3 CHRONIC RENAL FAILURE

In comparison with young adults, chronic renal failure (CRF) in old age is more commonly due to renovascular disease, obstructive nephropathy and malignancy (Table 10.4). The occurrence of nephrotic syndrome in elderly patients is usually due to membranous glomerulonephritis. This is often ominous because of the association of membranous glomerulonephritis with underlying malignancy (particularly gastrointestinal and bronchial carcinomas) and amyloidosis (associated with underlying myeloma, chronic lymphocytic leukaemia and Hodgkin's lymphoma). Certain drugs may cause chronic renal impairment in old age, particularly angiotensin-converting enzyme (ACE) inhibitors, non-steroidal anti-inflammatory agents and gold and penicillamine (for chronic rheumatoid disease), but renal function usually recovers when these nephrotoxins are stopped. In old age, the **anaemia associated with CRF** is less well tolerated, particularly in the presence of coexistent pathology, such as angina, cardiac failure, chronic respiratory disease and peripheral vascular disease.

Elderly patients with advanced CRF (plasma creatinine concentration $>300\,\mu mol/l$) and chronic anaemia (haemoglobin concentrations $<10\,g/dl$) should be considered for erythropoietin replacement, after exclusion of haematinic deficiencies and occult gastrointestinal blood loss. A trial of **epoietin alfa** 50–100 units/kg intravenously in dialysis patients (subcutaneously in non-dialysed CRF patients) three times per week is worthwhile, particularly when regular blood transfusion is poorly tolerated or is impractical for the patient.

Dietary **restriction of protein is no longer recommended** as part of CRF management, and **sodium restriction** is only necessary where the patient is hypertensive. In many elderly patients with CRF, **restriction of**

Table 10.4   Causes of chronic renal failure in old age

Obstructive uropathy (underlying prostatic disease)	Chronic pyelonephritis
	Multiple myeloma
Renovascular disease	Nephrocalcinosis
Chronic hypertension	Amyloidosis
Diabetic nephropathy	Glomerulonephritis (especially membranous)

potassium intake may not need to be as rigorous as in younger patients. This is because elderly uraemic patients are often malnourished and further potassium restriction may reduce nutritional intake. In addition, many elderly people have a relatively low sodium and potassium intake. Thus, dietary manipulation to suit the individual's needs is the best approach, rather than a uniformly rigid policy of sodium and potassium restriction where the patient's food intake declines because the patient does not find his/her diet appetizing. **Avoidance of potassium-sparing drugs** may be more important in preventing dangerous hyperkalaemia in elderly CRF patients, e.g. inadvertent prescribing of amiloride, triamterene and spironolactone in combination diuretics.

Hypertension usually warrants careful control, although the risk: benefit ratio from antihypertensive therapy in those aged over 80 is uncertain. Morbidity from **metabolic bone disease** due to the lack of hydroxylation of vitamin D in the kidney takes a higher toll in older patients, and is preventable with **1-α-hydroxycholecalciferol** (0.25–0.5 μg daily maintenance dose) and oral phosphate binders (e.g. aluminium hydroxide, calcium carbonate). **Pruritus** is another common and distressing problem for uraemic patients. **Emulsifying ointment 30%** and **liquid paraffin** added to bath water are helpful emollients for mild–moderate symptoms. For more severe symptoms, addition of suberythemal doses of **UVB irradiation** twice weekly may be helpful.

Dialysis has an important role to play in some elderly end-stage renal failure patients. With careful selection, elderly patients can remain well on dialysis programmes and often adjust better than younger patients to the restricted lifestyle that dialysis imposes. Elderly patients may be satisfactorily rehabilitated with haemodialysis or continuous ambulatory peritoneal dialysis (CAPD). However, CAPD requires considerable skill and dexterity, which may restrict its use in many elderly patients. In patients in whom haemodialysis is planned, the requirement for access to the circulation should be anticipated by fashioning of an **arteriovenous fistula** several months before the predicted requirement for dialysis. Such advance planning is particularly important in elderly patients who are at particular risk from overwhelming sepsis complicating the use of temporary vascular access catheters sited in large veins (e.g. internal jugular or subclavian lines).

Although **renal transplantation** is unusual in CRF patients over 70, it can be a highly valuable treatment option in selected older patients, with considerable improvement of qualify of life compared to long-term dialysis. Other advantages of transplantation in older patients include better graft tolerance with less need for intensive (and expensive) immunosuppression, favourable cost–benefit ratio compared to dialysis or conservative medical therapy. The overall state of the patient's health, rather than age, should be the overriding factor when considering patients for inclusion in transplant programmes. Major renal and iliac occlusive arterial disease and lower urinary tract pathology must be excluded prior to transplantation so that adequate allograft perfusion and drainage are ensured.

10.4 FEMALE GENITAL ATROPHY

Elderly women commonly suffer a variety of symptoms related to genital atrophy. These include vulval soreness, atrophic vaginitis and urethritis causing dysuria, urinary urgency and sometimes incontinence. Patients may notice bleeding following minor trauma such as wiping after micturition. Stress incontinence may be exacerbated by coexistent genital atrophy and sexually active women may complain of dyspareunia and postcoital bleeding. Physical examination reveals atrophy of vulval and vaginal tissues with inflammatory changes such as eroded, friable vaginal mucosa which has lost its typical rugose appearance. Sometimes, infective vaginal discharge occurs due to the combination of atrophic change and the loss of the normally acidic vaginal pH which prevents ingress of infecting organisms. Female genital atrophy is under-recognized and therefore undertreated because patients are often reticent about their symptoms or believe them to be 'just old age'. **Topical oestrogen** (dienoestrol 0.01% or conjugated oestrogen 0.625 mg/g cream or pessary) quickly relieves symptoms. In women with an intact uterus, the minimum effective amount should be applied. Locally applied oestrogen has similar efficacy to oral therapy at approximately a quarter of the dose. Treatment should be continued for several weeks after symptoms have settled or may be given continuously, in which case it is advisable to combine therapy with an oral progestogen for 10–14 days of each month to lessen the risk of endometrial hyperplasia and carcinoma.

10.5   SEXUAL DYSFUNCTION IN OLD AGE

Sexual activity is normal in old age. Although ageing tends to reduce the sexual response to some degree in men and women, these changes do not preclude satisfactory intercourse. However, erectile dysfunction affects about 25% of all men at age 65 and about half of all men at age 80. There are many underlying medical causes of erectile dysfunction, such as generalized arteriosclerotic vascular disease, cerebrovascular disease, spinal cord injury, peripheral neuropathy, diabetes mellitus, thyroid dysfunction, chronic renal failure, chronic liver disease and certain drugs (e.g. neuroleptics, antidepressants, anticholinergics, antihypertensives). Drugs, in particular, should be considered as possible causes of erectile dysfunction, since they are thought to contribute to the problem in about a quarter of all cases. Psychiatric disorders, particularly depression, anxiety and unresolved brief reactions, may also reduce libido and sexual function. Effective treatment of some of these disorders may improve or resolve the problem.

After exclusion of major endocrine causes of erectile dysfunction by screening of serum total and free testosterone, luteinizing hormone, thyroid function and blood glucose, **prostaglandin E_1 (alprostadil)** administered as an intracavernosal injection or urethral gel is useful as both a diagnostic and therapeutic manoeuvre. Men with sufficient penile arterial blood flow usually achieve an erection within 10–15 minutes after injection, which is sustained for 15–30 minutes. **Vacuum tumescent devices** may be tried before resorting to pharmacotherapy. If drug therapy is required, patients may be commenced on alprostadil urethral gel. **Sildenafil** (Viagra) is another drug that may have a role in the treatment of impotence. It is an orally active inhibitor of cyclic guanosine monophosphate in the corpus cavernosum which has been shown in recent trials to be significantly superior to placebo. It may produce side-effects of headache, flushing and dyspepsia. However, efficacy, safety and tolerability data in elderly men are awaited before its widespread prescription can be recommended. Nevertheless, its availability as a rapidly absorbed oral preparation may be an advantage over alprostadil. As a last resort, erectile dysfunction may be treated surgically by implantation of flexible metal or inflatable cavernal rods under local anaesthetic.

In females, intercourse may be painful as a result of oestrogen deficiency that results in vaginal dryness, mucosal atrophy and friability. **Local or systemic oestrogen** replacement therapy may restore satisfactory sexual intercourse in these circumstances (see section 10.4).

FURTHER READING

Baldessarre JS, Kaye D. Special problems of urinary tract infection in the elderly. *Med Clin North Am* 1991; 75:375–389.

DuBeau CE. Urinary incontinence. In: WB Abrams, MH Beers, R Berkow (eds). *The Merck Manual of Geriatrics*, 2nd edn. Merck Research Laboratories, Whitehouse Station, NJ, USA, 1995, pp 169–199.

Goldstein I, Lue TF, Padma-Nathan H et al. Oral sildenafil in the treatment of erectile dysfunction. Sildenafil Study Group. *N Engl J Med* 1998; 338:1397–1404.

Linet OI, Ogrinc FG. Efficacy and safety of intracavernosal alprostadil in men with erectile dysfunction. The Alprostadil Study Group. *N Engl J Med* 1996; 334:873–877.

Padma-Nathan H, Hellstrom WJ, Kaiser FE et al. Treatment of men with erectile dysfunction with transurethral alprostadil. Medicated Urethral System for Erection (MUSE) Study Group. *N Engl J Med* 1997; 336:1–7.

Royal College of Physicians of London. *Incontinence. Causes, Management and Provision of Services*. RCP, London, 1995.

Tobin GW. *Incontinence in the Elderly*. Edward Arnold, London, 1992.

Chapter 11

Eye and Ear Disorders

11.1 GLAUCOMA

Glaucoma is the single most important preventable cause of blindness in Western countries, and is predominantly a disorder of older people. It affects about 4% of people over 75 years and accounts for about 13% of all persons registered blind in the UK. Glaucoma is characterized by progressive optic disc cupping and constriction of the visual fields, eventually leading to tunnel vision and complete blindness. Intraocular pressure (IOP; normal range up to 20 mmHg) is usually but not always raised in glaucoma. There are two common types of glaucoma: primary open-angle glaucoma, which is a chronic condition, and closed-angle glaucoma, which usually presents as an acute ophthalmic emergency.

The cause of **primary open-angle glaucoma** is unclear. Risk factors include affected first degree relatives, myopia, hypertension, diabetes mellitus and African-Caribbean ethnic origin. In this condition, there is an imbalance between aqueous humour production by the ciliary body in the posterior chamber and drainage of fluid through the trabecular meshwork of the anterior chamber into the canal of Schlemm. Primary open-angle glaucoma does not usually cause symptoms in the early stages, so screening of those at higher risk (i.e. elderly people) is important and worthwhile. The combination of fundoscopy, tonometry and visual field examination is the best approach, and is carried out by optometrists as part of a sight test. The aim of treatment is to prevent visual loss by reducing IOP by approximately 30%. Intraocular pressure levels may need to be less than 10 mmHg in some patients to arrest visual deterioration. Raised IOP may be reduced by either suppressing the production of aqueous humour or improving its outflow, or both. Aqueous humour production is reduced by topical beta-blockers, carbonic anhydrase inhibitors (topical or systemic) and the topical alpha-2-adrenergic agonist, brimonidine.

Topical beta-blockers are the most widely used agents (e.g. **timolol**, **levobunolol**) and most block beta-1 and beta-2 receptors. Some systemic absorption occurs and may cause significant problems in patients in whom beta-blockers are contraindicated, e.g. patients with concurrent chronic obstructive pulmonary disease (COPD) or cardiac failure. Although the cardioselective beta-blocker, **betaxolol**, may cause fewer pulmonary side-effects, it should still be used with caution in patients with COPD. Timolol 0.25–0.5% and carteolol 1–2% are the most widely used preparations, usually applied twice daily to both eyes. Carbonic anhydrase inhibitors (e.g. acetazolamide) are prescribed less commonly for primary open-angle glaucoma nowadays, because of better tolerated, more effective topical agents. Recently, however, a topical carbonic anhydrase inhibitor (**dorzolamide** 2% three times daily) has been shown to be as effective as topical timolol 0.5% and betaxolol 0.5% when given over a 1-year period. However, topical dorzolamide may be associated with adverse side-effects of headache, bitter taste, ocular discomfort, blurred vision and watering eyes. **Brimonidine** 0.2% twice daily is a useful second-line treatment in conjunction with either topical beta-blockers or dorzolamide.

Aqueous humour outflow is facilitated by topical agents that induce ciliary muscle contraction (e.g. **pilocarpine**) or enhance flow through the trabecular meshwork (e.g. **adrenaline** and its prodrug, **dipivefrine**). Pilocarpine may be applied as eye drops or as a gel. It may cause blurred vision and headache as a result of ciliary muscle spasm. Adrenaline and dipivefrine may be absorbed systemically and should be used with caution in patients with hypertension and heart disease. A new prostaglandin F2α analogue, **latanoprost**, has recently been introduced. It works by increasing uveoscleral outflow of aqueous humour and is mainly used in those patients unable to tolerate or poorly responsive to other treatments. It is used once daily at night and should be administered under ophthalmic supervision. It may cause darkening of the iris and eyelashes, ocular irritation, conjunctival hyperaemia and sometimes erosions.

Surgical treatment with a trabeculoplasty is indicated in patients whose IOP remains raised or who have deteriorating visual fields despite maximal topical drug therapy. The aim of the procedure is to create drainage of aqueous humour between the anterior chamber and the subconjunctival sac, thereby reducing IOP. If surgery is contraindicated or must be postponed, laser trabeculoplasty is an alternative to surgery that is well tolerated, quick and suitable for elderly patients who cannot instil eye drops. It can also be used to complement medical therapy. Surgery is more effective than laser therapy and is being used more widely and earlier, particularly in those presenting with high IOPs.

Acute closed-angle glaucoma is an ophthalmic emergency that usually presents with severe supraorbital pain, blurred vision, headache, nausea and vomiting. The patient is distressed, has a painful red eye, a hazy cornea, and a dilated unreactive pupil. The other eye is at risk of developing a similar acute episode. **Topical pilocarpine and intravenous acetazolamide** 250–500 mg are used to reduce IOP whilst arrangements are being made for urgent ophthalmological referral for **laser iridotomy**. Laser therapy is recommended for both eyes in view of the high risk of acute glaucoma in the unaffected eye.

In susceptible people, glaucoma may be precipitated or exacerbated by certain drugs, principally anticholinergics (including tricyclic antidepressants), glucocorticoids and topical mydiatics. In cases of known glaucoma, these drugs should be avoided, if possible.

11.2 CATARACTS

Cataracts are common in old age and are often incidental findings on physical examination that do not cause symptoms. Impaired vision from early cataracts may be helped by correction of associated myopic defects with a change of spectacle lenses. If vision fails to improve, or if a patient's vision no longer meets his/her needs, surgical cataract removal is indicated. This procedure is usually performed under local anaesthesia and involves phakoemulsification of the nucleus and cortex of the lens, leaving the posterior capsule intact. The focus is restored by intraocular lens implantation. Where this is not possible, a continuous wear contact lens may be fitted. Cataracts should be removed before they cause severe loss of vision, particularly since visual impairment is a common cause of accidents in elderly people. Ninety-five per cent of those with visual impairment due to cataract report improved vision following extraction.

11.3   AGE-RELATED MACULAR DEGENERATION

Age-related macular degeneration (ARMD) is now the leading cause of blindness in persons over 65 in Western countries. The aetiology and pathophysiology of ARMD are unclear, and ARMD is likely to become an even greater public health problem over the next 30–40 years, given the projected substantial increases in the numbers of persons who are most at risk, i.e. those over 75. There is no known effective preventive or curative therapy. The majority of patients have dry, atrophic retinal changes characterized by pigment atrophy and dispersion, and a build-up of colloid bodies (drusen) beneath the retina. A slow deterioration of reading vision results. 'Wet' exudative macular degeneration can develop, characterized by complaints of distortion of straight lines. A few patients may be helped by laser photocoagulation when there is subretinal neovascularization away from the fovea that presents a high risk of acute macular haemorrhage and rapid deterioration of vision. In most cases, however, the pathology is beneath the macula and is untreatable. Sufferers may be helped by a variety of low vision aids as well as being registered partially-sighted or blind, as appropriate, to ensure statutory entitlements and services from appropriate institutional and voluntary agencies (e.g. the Royal National Institute for the Blind in the UK).

11.4   MISCELLANEOUS OPHTHALMIC DISORDERS OF OLD AGE

Sudden loss of vision in one eye is a clinical emergency requiring expert ophthalmological assessment without delay. The major causes in older people are central retinal artery occlusion (CRAO), central retinal vein occlusion (CRVO), acute closed-angle glaucoma, ischaemic optic neuropathy (usually giant cell arteritis) and transient ischaemic attacks from embolic episodes. The acutely ischaemic retina from CRAO looks characteristically pale, retinal artery branches are less conspicuous and the fovea has a 'cherry-red' appearance. The retinal circulation needs to be re-established within about 1 hour if vision is to be saved. The ophthalmologist may restore complete or partial reperfusion with ocular paracentesis as a first-line treatment. CRVO causes visual loss varying from 6/18 to detection of hand movements only. The retinal veins are engorged, and there are widespread blot haemorrhages. Urgent ophthalmic referral is needed as some patients require laser treatment to prevent the blinding complication of neovascular glaucoma. If the cause of CRAO is probably thromboembolic, thrombolysis may be tried and the patient investigated for cardiac and carotid disease. If there is suspicion of giant cell arteritis, the patients should receive immediate high-dose steroid therapy (prednisolone 60–80 mg).

Xerophthalmia (dry eyes) in old age most commonly results from idiopathic keratoconjunctivitis sicca, where there is degeneration of lacrimal gland tissue and failure of tear production. Patients complain of gritty, painful eyes. **Artificial tears** (e.g. methylcellulose, hydroxyethylcellulose, hypromellose) applied frequently give good symptom relief.

Ectropion and **entropion** are most commonly seen in old people. They may be associated with painful, red, discharging eyes (particularly entropion). Entropion causes the eyelashes to abrade the cornea and requires corrective surgery. Ectropion may be misdiagnosed as conjunctivitis, thereby exposing patients to unnecessary topical antibiotics (usually chloramphenicol). If necessary, ectropion may be corrected by a simple plastic surgery procedure.

11.5 EAR PROBLEMS

Impacted cerumen (earwax) is a common problem in older people who complain of deafness. Often, the elderly people are unaware of external auditory canal obstruction and every person noted to be deaf should have otoscopy to exclude this easily remediable problem. A variety of cerumenolytics have been used over recent decades, such as vegetable oils, 5% hydrogen peroxide, 5% sodium bicarbonate and docusate sodium, all of which help soften the cerumen but none of which has been shown to be a clearly superior treatment. Cerumen should be softened for a few days with 5% sodium bicarbonate (cheap and less messy), before attempting clearance, with gentle ear syringing (water at body temperature) or instrumental removal using an ear speculum. If there is any suspicion of tympanic membrane perforation, syringing should be avoided because of the risk of inducing otitis media.

Deafness is the major communication disorder of old age. The physiological ageing process results in some hearing loss in the high frequencies (presbycusis) but this is seldom a cause of auditory handicap. On formal testing, about 50% of elderly people have hearing impairment, of whom half feel able to cope well and do not feel they need hearing aids. Approximately 20–25% of those elderly people who would benefit from a hearing aid actually have and use one properly. All deaf elderly people require a detailed audiological evaluation to establish the type of deafness and whether they can be rehabilitated (e.g. with a behind-the-ear hearing aid). Traditional **microphonic hearing aids** have been improved upon in recent years, with the introduction of the digitally programmable hearing aid, which further improves speech clarity. Audibility of sound from televisions and radios may be enhanced by use of headphones plugged into the listening jack present in most modern sets.

Many frail deaf people cannot manage conventional hearing aids because it requires good visual acuity and manual dexterity to operate and maintain most behind-the-ear devices. A simple checklist helps correct most malfunctions, and it is helpful if relatives and carers are familiar with this (Table 11.1). If there are still problems, elderly patients may cope very well with simpler microphonic amplification devices ('Communicators'), clipped to a shirt or blouse, and connected to an earpiece or to headphones. The ever decreasing size and conspicuousness of headphones make this option more acceptable for patients and carers. The body-worn devices are the most powerful sound amplifying hearing aids available and may be easier for many elderly people to adjust than the behind-the-ear device. **Bone-conduction hearing aids** may help in some cases where in-the-ear air-conduction hearing aids are

Table 11.1 Checklist of easily correctable malfunctions of hearing aids

Problem	Solution
(1) Cerumen blockage of earpiece	Dislodge cerumen with dry cloth or needle.
(2) No sound amplification	Make sure microphone is switched on ('M'). Check volume control (should be feedback squeal on maximum volume). Change batteries if problem not resolved.
(3) Cannot hear telephone speech	Make sure dial turned to 'T' (telecoil).

unsuitable, e.g. chronic otorrhoea. They conduct sound through the mastoid bone directly to the auditory nerve by means of direct apposition with the mastoid and are worn as head sets. Hearing aids represent only one component of auditory rehabilitation. The occupational therapist has an important role in helping deaf persons to deal with the wide variety of handicaps resulting from deafness, e.g. adjustments to telephones, home security systems, fire alarms, etc.

Deafness may be drug-induced, e.g. high-dose aminoglycosides, loop diuretics, salicylates and quinine. Aminoglycosides may be particularly toxic in high plasma concentrations, often resulting in permanent ototoxic damage in elderly people with pre-existent presbycusis and more established hearing loss.

FURTHER READING

Corrado OJ. Hearing aids. In: G Mulley (ed). *Everyday Aids and Appliances*. British Medical Journal Publications, London, 1989, pp 1–8.

Diamond JP. Systemic adverse effects of topical ophthalmic agents. Implications for older patients. *Drugs Aging* 1997; 11:352–360.

Fisch L, Brooks DN. Disorders of hearing. In: JC Brocklehurst, RC Tallis, HM Fillit (eds). *Textbook of Gerontology and Geriatric Medicine*, 4th edn. Churchill Livingstone, Edinburgh, 1992, pp 480–493.

Tee Khaw P. Glaucoma 2: Developments in treatment of primary open-angle glaucoma. *Prescriber J* 1997; 37:40–45.

Chapter 12

Haematological Disorders

12.1 IRON DEFICIENCY ANAEMIA

Iron deficiency anaemia is the commonest cause of anaemia in every country of the world and results in a microcytic, hypochromic anaemia. Patients may present with pallor, dyspnoea, headache and fatigue. In addition, they may develop angular stomatitis, a painless glossitis and occasionally brittle, rigid or spoon nails (koilonychia), dysphagia due to pharyngeal webs and unusual dietary cravings (pica).

12.1.1 Causes

Chronic blood loss from the gastrointestinal tract is the commonest cause of iron deficiency anaemia in the elderly. Blood loss from pelvic, renal or bladder tumours may also result in iron deficiency. Inadequate intake of iron rarely is the sole cause of anaemia and even when the diet is poor the patient should be fully investigated for blood loss. Despite this, dietary deficiency of iron is a genuine entity and is often underestimated, particularly in elderly people who consume large amounts of tea. The tannic acid in tea reduces the absorption of dietary iron.

12.1.2 Diagnosis

The diagnosis is made by the finding of a hypochromic microcytic anaemia on the blood film. Pencil cells are frequently seen. Thrombocytosis may occur if the patient is bleeding but is more often secondary to the iron deficiency state itself. In otherwise healthy people, a serum ferritin of $<100\,\mu g/l$ is diagnostic. This is associated with an iron saturation (serum iron/total iron binding capacity) of $<15\%$ except in patients with inflammatory, infective or liver disease whose iron saturation may be >15% despite an iron deficiency state.

12.1.3 Investigation

In elderly men and women gastrointestinal blood loss is the main cause of iron deficiency anaemia and the exact site is sought from the clinical history, physical and rectal examination and by appropriate use of upper gastrointestinal endoscopy, sigmoidoscopy, colonoscopy and imaging. Rarely a coeliac axis angiogram is needed to demonstrate angio-dysplasia.

12.1.4 Treatment

The underlying cause is treated as far as is possible and oral iron is started. The best preparation is **ferrous sulphate** given two or three times daily (67 mg iron in each 200 mg (anhydrous) tablet). It may also be given as a syrup if tablets are difficult to swallow. Absorption is helped by giving it in the fasting state, or with vitamin C containing foods such as citrus fruits, but adverse effects such as nausea, abdominal pain, diarrhoea or constipation are less common if it is given with meals. Preparations with a lower iron content, e.g. ferrous gluconate (37 mg iron per 300 mg tablet), may also help. Enteric-coated or sustained-release preparations should be avoided because the iron is often released distal to the site of absorption in the duodenum and they are relatively expensive. Therapy should be given for 4–6 months in order to correct the anaemia and replenish iron stores. The haemoglobin should rise by 2 g/dl every 3 weeks. Failure of response has several causes which should be considered before parenteral iron is used (Table 12.1).

Table 12.1 Failure of response to oral iron

Continuing blood loss
Poor compliance
Mixed deficiency—associated B_{12} or folate deficiency
Wrong diagnosis—malignancy or inflammation
Malabsorption—rare
Slow release preparation—releases iron in lower small intestine

Occasionally, however, intramuscular iron may be necessary when patients cannot tolerate oral preparations because of gastric irritation or severe constipation or where there is poor compliance. Usually this is not necessary if lower doses of oral iron given as a syrup are combined with vitamin C.

12.2 MEGALOBLASTIC ANAEMIAS

This is a group of anaemias in which the erythroblasts in the bone marrow show a characteristic abnormality with delayed maturation of the nucleus due to defective DNA synthesis. The commonest causes are vitamin B_{12} and folate deficiency. Macrocytic anaemia without megaloblastic change may be due to alcoholism, liver disease, hypothyroidism, reticulocytosis, cytotoxic drugs, myelomatosis and myelodysplasia.

12.2.1 Folate Deficiency

Folate cannot be synthesized in the body and is ingested in liver, green vegetables and yeast. It is needed in the body for a variety of biochemical reactions including DNA synthesis. Low serum and red cell levels occur more often in elderly than in young people and deficiency is most often due to a poor intake of folate alone or in combination with increased folate utilization or malabsorption (Table 12.2). In addition, anti-folate

Table 12.2 Causes of folate deficiency in the elderly

Poor nutrition, particularly institutionalized, demented or ill patients

Malabsorption
   Partial gastrectomy, extensive jejunal resection or Crohn's disease

Excess utilization
   Malignant disease: carcinoma, lymphoma, myeloma
   Inflammatory disease: rheumatoid arthritis, psoriasis

Drugs
   Antiepileptics, sulphasalazine

Alcoholism

drugs such as phenytoin, trimethoprim and methotrexate may cause megaloblastic anaemia.

12.2.2 Vitamin B$_{12}$ Deficiency

This vitamin is found in foods of animal origin such as liver, fish and dairy produce but does not occur in fruit, cereals or vegetables unless these have been contaminated by bacteria. Following ingestion it is bound with intrinsic factor produced by gastric parietal cells and this complex is absorbed in the distal ileum via specific surface receptors for intrinsic factor. B$_{12}$ is a coenzyme for two biochemical reactions in the body involving methylation of homocysteine to methionine and conversion of coenzyme A (CoA) to succinyl CoA. In Western countries, B$_{12}$ deficiency is usually due to autoimmune pernicious anaemia. Much less commonly it may be caused by veganism in which the diet lacks B$_{12}$, gastrectomy or small intestinal lesions (Table 12.3).

12.2.3 Pernicious Anaemia

This is caused by an autoimmune atrophy of the stomach resulting in achlorhydria and reduced or absent secretion of intrinsic factor. The disease tends to occur in families and is associated with blood group A, blue eyes, early greying and an increased incidence of carcinoma of the stomach. Ninety per cent of patients have parietal cell antibodies in the

Table 12.3 Causes of vitamin B$_{12}$ deficiency

Nutritional—especially vegans

Malabsorption

Gastric causes
  Pernicious anaemia
  Total or partial gastrectomy

Intestinal causes
  Blind loop, stricture
  Ileal resection
  Crohn's disease

serum and 50% have a type I or blocking antibody to intrinsic factor which inhibits binding of vitamin B_{12}, and 35% of patients show a type II or precipitating antibody to intrinsic factor which inhibits its ileal binding site. Intrinsic factor antibodies are virtually specific for pernicious anaemia whereas parietal cell antibodies are rather non-specific.

12.2.4 Clinical Features of Megaloblastic Anaemia

Patients present with symptoms and signs of anaemia. They may be mildly jaundiced due to excessive breakdown of haemoglobin caused by defective erythropoiesis.

12.2.5 Vitamin B_{12} Neuropathy (Subacute Combined Degeneration of the Cord)

Severe B_{12} deficiency may cause a progressive symmetrical neuropathy affecting peripheral sensory nerves and posterior and pyramidal tract columns, mainly in the lower limbs. Rarely optic atrophy or psychiatric symptoms are present. Central nervous system involvement requires more intensive replacement therapy and recovery is generally poor.

12.2.6 Diagnosis

Patients present with a macrocytic anaemia. The reticulocyte count is low in relation to the degree of anaemia and the white cell and platelet count may also be reduced. The bone marrow is hypercellular and the erythrocytes are large with failure of nuclear maturation. Serum B_{12} is low, serum folate normal or raised and red cell folate normal or low in megaloblastic anaemia or neurological impairment due to B_{12} deficiency. Both the serum and red cell folate are low in megaloblastic anaemia due to folate deficiency and the latter must be low in order to make the diagnosis. Combined deficiencies may be difficult to identify but haematological response to specific therapy is helpful, using $1\,\mu g$ B_{12} or $100\,\mu g$ folate daily. Large doses of folate ($5\,mg$ daily) may aggravate the neuropathy of B_{12} deficiency and should therefore not be given alone unless B_{12} deficiency has been excluded. To test for the cause of B_{12} deficiency the Schilling test may be performed but in practice is seldom used clinically. If the patient is intrinsic factor antibody positive, vitamin B_{12} injection therapy is started and haematological parameters are monitored. Vitamin B_{12} malabsorption may also result from small bowel bacterial overgrowth. If this is suspected, empirical antibiotic therapy is given for 8–12 weeks. If this fails to improve serum vitamin B_{12} levels a Schilling test may be useful, to elucidate the cause of vitamin B_{12} malabsorption.

12.2.7   Treatment

For vitamin B_{12} deficiency, intramuscular hydroxocobalamin (1 mg) is given daily for one week. Then 1 mg is given weekly for one month or until haemoglobin is normal. After that, 1 mg is given every 3 months. Folate deficiency is treated with 5 mg orally per day until the red cell folate and haemoglobin concentrations are normal and dietary intake is assured. Continuous folate therapy is indicated during long-term phenytoin, methotrexate or cotrimoxazole therapy. The haemoglobin concentration should rise by 2 to 3 g/dl every fortnight and white cell and platelet counts should become normal in 7 to 10 days. Oral potassium supplements may rarely be needed if hypokalaemia occurs during the initial haematological response. Blood transfusion should be avoided if at all possible since it may cause circulatory overload, and exacerbate bone marrow suppression.

12.3   ANAEMIA OF CHRONIC DISEASE

Patients with a variety of chronic inflammatory and malignant diseases may present with a normochromic (or mildly hypochromic), normocytic (or microcytic) anaemia with reduced serum iron and total iron binding capacity and normal or raised serum ferritin. These anaemias are primarily disorders of iron re-utilization and marrow stores are normal. The anaemia is only corrected by successful treatment of the underlying disease but in rheumatoid arthritis or myeloma a partial response to recombinant erythropoietin may be obtained. The causes are

Table 12.4   Causes of the anaemia of chronic disease

Chronic inflammatory disease
Infectious: tuberculosis, osteomyelitis, pneumonia, bacterial endocarditis
Non-infectious: rheumatoid arthritis, systemic lupus erythematosus, sarcoid, Crohn's
disease, polymyalgia rheumatica

Malignant disease
Carcinoma, lymphoma, sarcoma, myeloma

---

listed in Table 12.4. In many cases the anaemia may be complicated by iron or folate deficiency, renal failure, bone marrow infiltration or hypersplenism.

12.4   BLOOD TRANSFUSION

12.4.1   Indications for Blood Transfusion

Whole blood is used for treating acute blood loss following trauma or surgery and acute gastrointestinal or uterine haemorrhage. For acute blood loss of up to 2 units the use of plasma-reduced cells plus electrolyte solution is recommended. Packed red cells are the treatment of choice in chronically anaemic patients who require transfusion because of symptoms of anaemia. In these patients the haemoglobin level alone is not a good guide to transfusion requirement because of the wide variation in cardiovascular adaptation. In elderly patients, diuretic therapy may be given simultaneously and the transfusion must be administered slowly to avoid circulatory overload. In the majority of patients with deficiency anaemias appropriate treatment with iron, folate or vitamin B_{12} is sufficient and transfusions are seldom required.

12.4.2   Complications of Blood Transfusion

Before blood transfusion, compatibility between donor red cell antigens and the recipient's plasma antibodies must be ensured. Approximately 400 red blood cell group antigens have been described but the ABO and rhesus antigens are by far the most clinically significant. During transfusion individuals who lack a particular blood group antigen may produce antibodies to it and potentially fatal haemolytic reactions may occur. To avoid this the blood group of the patient is determined before transfusion and the serum screened for atypical antibodies. Blood of the same ABO and rhesus group as the recipient is used. Red cells from each donor unit are tested against the patient's serum (cross matching). On the rare occasions where the urgency of the clinical situation does not allow time for grouping and cross matching, group O rhesus negative blood may be transfused.

12.4.3   Haemolytic Transfusion Reactions

Haemolytic transfusion reactions may be immediate or delayed. Immediate life-threatening reactions associated with massive intravascular haemolysis are the result of complement activating IgM or IgG antibodies, e.g. to ABO groups, and are usually due to clinical errors. The severity of the reaction depends on the recipient's titre of antibody. Delayed reactions are caused when the pretransfusion level of an antibody is too low to be detected during the cross match. The patient is then reimmunized during transfusion and there may follow a delayed transfusion reaction with accelerated clearance of red cells leading to anaemia and mild jaundice.

The clinical features of a major haemolytic transfusion reaction include urticaria, lumbar pain, flushing, headache, precordial chest pain, shortness of breath, rigors, pyrexia and a fall in blood pressure which may occur at any stage during the transfusion or 1–2 hours afterwards. Jaundice, haemoglobinuria, disseminated intravascular coagulation and acute renal failure may subsequently occur. If a patient develops features suggestive of a severe transfusion reaction the transfusion should be stopped immediately and investigations for blood group incompatibility and bacterial contamination of the blood initiated. Initial treatment is with intravenous saline, hydrocortisone 100 mg and an antihistamine (e.g. chlorpheniramine 10 mg). Subcutaneous or intramuscular adrenaline (0.5–1 ml, 1 : 1000) is reserved for patients in severe shock. Acute renal failure is managed in the usual way.

Table 12.5 Complications of blood transfusions

Haemolytic reactions
Reactions due to infected blood
Allergic reactions to white cells, platelets or proteins
Pyrogenic reactions to plasma proteins or HLA antibodies
Circulatory overload
Air embolus
Thrombophlebitis
Hyperkalaemia
Citrate toxicity
Clotting abnormalities after massive transfusion
Transmission of infection

The causes of other transfusion reactions are listed in Table 12.5. Reactions to white cell antibodies may be prevented by giving leuco-cyte-depleted (filtered) packed cells. Hypersensitivity allergic reactions to plasma proteins may be prevented by giving washed or frozen red cells. Most cases of post-transfusion hepatitis are due to hepatitis B or C. HIV may also be transmitted in cellular and plasma components of blood. In order to reduce the risk, all blood donations are screened for hepatitis B and HIV and donors for hepatitis C.

12.5 CHRONIC MYELOID LEUKAEMIA

Chronic myeloid leukaemia (CML) is most common in middle age but is also seen in the elderly. Patients present with symptoms of anaemia, weight loss, anorexia and night sweats. Easy bruising or haemorrhage may occur due to abnormal platelet function. Hyperuricaemia may cause gout and renal impairment. Splenomegaly is common and may be massive. A leucocytosis $>50\times10^9$/l with mature white cells and basophils in the peripheral blood is typical. Philadelphia (Ph) chromosome is seen on cytogenetic analysis of blood or marrow.

12.5.1 Treatment

The treatment of CML has become more complicated in recent years. Previously, most patients were treated with busulphan as long as they remained in the chronic phase of their disease. If they became resistant to busulphan they were switched to hydroxyurea. However, since the discovery that **interferon**-α could induce remissions in up to 80% of patients with CML, this has become the agent of first choice. Its use is limited by considerable dose-related toxicity including nausea, influenza-like symptoms, lethargy, ocular side-effects and depression. Myelosuppression may also occur, as may hypersensitivity reaction, rashes and confusion, particularly with high doses in elderly patients. Bone marrow transplantation is the only way of curing the disease but is usually applicable only to younger patients. Splenic irradiation is reserved for patients whose splenic enlargement is not responsive to chemotherapy and causes clinical problems such as pain and anaemia. Splenectomy is rarely performed in CML.

12.5.2   Prognosis

Most patients pursue a course of good health over several years which is in marked contrast to the rapid and striking deterioration when transformation to acute myeloid leukaemia occurs. Survival is then measured in weeks or months.

12.6   CHRONIC LYMPHOCYTIC LEUKAEMIA

This occurs mostly in elderly people and presents with lymphadenopathy, anaemia, thrombocytopenia and hepatosplenomegaly. It is the most common leukaemia after the age of 60. It is frequently diagnosed on routine blood testing with a raised white cell count ($>15–300 \times 10^9$/l) and up to 99% of the white cells on the film appearing as lymphocytes. The disease has been divided into stages A, B and C based on the degree of organ involvement (nodes, liver and spleen), haemoglobin and platelet levels. These stages correlate with different prognoses. Stage A patients usually survive for many years while those with stage C disease will only live for about 18 months. Fifty per cent of patients will have stage A disease at diagnosis.

12.6.1 Treatment

Patients often have a good prognosis so treatment is reserved for those with symptoms due to bone marrow failure, lymph node involvement, hypersplenism, autoimmune haemolytic anaemia or thrombocytopenia. Treatment options include corticosteroids, alkylating agents (chlorambucil or cyclophosphamide), radiotherapy or combination chemotherapy.

12.6.2 Prognosis

Most patients survive 3–5 years but patients with slowly progressive diseases may survive for more than 10 years.

12.7 MYELODYSPLASTIC SYNDROMES

The myelodysplastic syndromes (MDS) are characterized by chronic anaemia, leucopenia and thrombocytopenia with normocellular or hypercellular marrow. The prevalence is about 1 : 500 in people over 60 years. The spectrum of morphological appearances is very wide and the natural history of these disorders varies widely, ranging from low to high leukaemic conversion rates and good to poor prognosis. MDS are classified into five categories according to the number of blast cells in the bone marrow and peripheral blood and other characteristics such as the presence of ringed sideroblasts in the bone marrow. The categories are:

   (i) refractory anaemia
  (ii) refractory anaemia with ringed sideroblasts
 (iii) refractory anaemia with excess blasts (RAEB)
  (iv) chronic myelomonocytic leukaemia
   (v) RAEB in transformation.

12.7.1 Clinical Features

The majority of patients develop symptoms related to anaemia, leucopenia and thrombocytopenia. The blood film often shows a macrocytic pattern with reticulocytopenia. There is no specific marker for MDS and the diagnosis is made by examination of the bone marrow which shows dysplasia with qualitative abnormalities such as ringed sideroblasts and increased numbers of blast cells. The pancytopenia has to be distinguished from treatable conditions such as B_{12} and folate deficiency and other causes of bone marrow infiltration. Death usually results from pancytopenia or acute leukaemic transformation that is resistant to conventional chemotherapy. Prognosis is determined by karyotype abnormalities of the malignant clone.

12.7.2   Treatment

Much of the treatment of elderly MDS patients is supportive, with treatment of infective episodes by broad-spectrum antibiotics and anaemia by transfusion of filtered blood and platelets when required. Bone marrow transplantation is the treatment of choice in young adults but is not appropriate in the elderly. In patients who are clinically stable and have criteria indicating a good prognosis, treatment is generally not started but they are kept under close follow-up. Occasionally corticosteroids may be useful. For elderly patients the use of aggressive chemotherapy is associated with a high complication rate and no improvement in survival. It is therefore not usually recommended. Therapy with marrow cell line differentiating agents is being explored. Iron overload may be a problem with repeated, frequent transfusions so serum ferritin should be monitored. Subcutaneous desferrioxamine is rarely given because it is inconvenient and the patient usually dies of MDS complications other than iron overload, or intercurrent diseases.

12.8   MULTIPLE MYELOMA

Multiple myeloma is a malignant proliferation of plasma cells and plasma cell precursors. The major clinical manifestations result from accumulation of these cells and the characteristic protein secreted from them. There is an increasing incidence with age and the median age at diagnosis is 69 years.

Table 12.6 Mechanisms which result in the clinical manifestations of multiple myeloma

Direct tumour growth causing replacement of normal structures
Accumulation of immunoglobulin chains causing hyperviscosity and amyloid
Release of cytokines by the plasma cells resulting in bone resorption

12.8.1 Clinical Features

Many of the clinical features are due to one of three mechanisms (Table 12.6).

Skeletal Complications

Bone pain is the commonest complaint in newly diagnosed patients, occurring in 60–70%. Multiple osteolytic lesions throughout the skeleton are typical but pathological fractures and generalized osteopenia are also common. Skeletal survey remains the best way to determine the extent of bone disease. Magnetic resonance imaging (MRI) is useful for detecting early bone lesions in selected cases or in evaluating cord compression. The loss of bone that occurs in multiple myeloma is secondary to excessive bone resorption from activated osteoclasts with normal or reduced bone formation.

Hypercalcaemia

The clinical manifestations of hypercalcaemia may be subtle in the elderly (see Chapter 6). Although bone resorption increases the risk of hypercalcaemia, renal insufficiency and dehydration are usually contributing factors. Inactivity due to bone pain also adds to the process.

Anaemia

A normochromic, normocytic (or macrocytic) anaemia is present at diagnosis in two-thirds of patients and is associated with a markedly raised erythrocyte sedimentation rate.

Renal Failure

Up to 50% of patients have renal failure at diagnosis. Many of these cases are reversible with rehydration and treatment of the myeloma but irreversible renal failure is a poor prognostic factor. Most commonly renal failure is due to hypercalcaemia and Bence Jones proteinuria, which account for over 90% of cases of renal dysfunction. Light chains can precipitate in the tubules leading to obstruction and dilatation. Other manifestations include Fanconi's syndrome, plasma cell infiltration, amyloid infection and hyperuricaemia.

Amyloid and Hyperviscosity

Myeloma-associated amyloid is the result of deposition of immunoglobulin light chains in susceptible organs such as the kidneys, myocardium, gut and peripheral nerves. The amyloid is easily detected in tissue biopsies of bone marrow, abdominal skin, kidney or rectal mucosa with the use of Congo red stain. Manifestations of hyperviscosity include mucosal bleeding, retinopathy, neurological changes (TIAs and stroke) and congestive cardiac failure, and are related to sludging of blood flow in the microcirculation. Patients with hypertension or diabetes are more susceptible to hyperviscosity. It is particularly common in IgM paraprotein as seen in Waldenström's macroglobulinaemia.

Hypogammaglobulinaemia and Infection

Normal immunoglobulins are reduced in patients with myeloma and this together with steroid treatment leaves patients susceptible to infection.

12.8.2   Diagnosis and Staging

The usual clue to the diagnosis of multiple myeloma is the detection of a monoclonal band in the serum. However, many of these patients will not have myeloma but benign variants, i.e. MGUS—monoclonal gammopathy of undetermined significance. Unless these patients develop

Table 12.7   Diagnostic criteria for multiple myeloma

Two out of the following three criteria are needed for diagnosis:
(1) Serum or urine paraprotein
(2) Lytic bone lesions
(3) Marrow plasmacytosis

myeloma (which has a 17% incidence over 20 years) they do not require treatment. Table 12.7 shows the diagnostic criteria for multiple myeloma.

12.8.3   Treatment

Multiple myeloma remains a difficult disease to treat because of its marked resistance to chemotherapy. With conventional treatment not all patients respond and even in responding patients complete remissions are rare and relapse is inevitable. Patients with asymptomatic or equivocal myeloma (i.e. with normal haemoglobin, normal renal function and no bone lesions and with only a modest increase in plasma cells in the marrow) should not be treated at this stage but need careful follow-up. Although there are several treatment options for patients with unequivocal myeloma, for those over 70 a single oral alkylating agent such as **melphalan** is as effective as any other treatment. Intermittent oral melphalan has been shown to prolong survival to between 2 and 3 years. The inclusion of prednisolone in addition to melphalan has never been shown to improve long-term survival but improves the speed of response and reduces myelotoxicity. With this type of treatment 50–60% of patients will respond usually over a period of 3–6 months and will reach a stable plateau. Treatment is usually stopped at this stage since giving further chemotherapy does not prolong the duration of the remission and may cause drug resistance.

Radiotherapy is useful as an adjunct to chemotherapy when a specific area needs rapid treatment to reduce pain, to treat cord compression or to prevent fracture through a large lytic lesion. If fracture has occurred it may be treated with intramedullary pins and radiotherapy.

Bisphosphonates are used for the treatment of hypercalcaemia in myeloma but will also reduce the progression of bone disease (see Chapter 8).

12.8.4   Prognosis

The average survival is still only 2 to 3 years.

12.9 MYELOPROLIFERATIVE DISORDERS

Polycythaemia rubra vera, essential thrombocythaemia and myelofibrosis are known as the non-leukaemic myeloproliferative disorders.

12.9.1 Polycythaemia Rubra Vera

This is caused by an overproduction of red blood cells, platelets and granulocytes. It occurs in elderly patients and the clinical features result from hyperviscosity and hypermetabolism (Table 12.8). The haemoglobin, haematocrit and red cell count are all increased. A neutrophil leucocytosis and raised platelet count is seen in about 50% of patients. The bone marrow is hypercellular with prominent megakaryocytes. It must be differentiated from causes of secondary polycythaemia such as hypoxia, cigarette smoking, cyanotic heart disease, renal cystic disease, cerebellar haemangioma, renal and hepatocellular carcinoma.

Treatment is aimed at maintaining a normal blood count with packed cell volume at 45% and platelet count below 400×10^9/l. **Venesection** is useful, particularly in those with mild disease although it does not control the platelet count. Cytotoxic chemotherapy with **busulphan** or **hydroxyurea** is indicated for more severe disease and reduces the risk of thrombosis. Such therapy needs close supervision with regular blood counts. **Phosphorus-32 (^{32}P)** is an effective myelosuppressive with a

Table 12.8   Clinical features of polycythemia rubra vera

Headaches
Pruritus after hot bath
Dyspnoea
Blurred vision
Plethoric appearance—ruddy cyanosis, conjunctival suffusion,
    retinal venous engorgement
Splenomegaly
Haemorrhage
Thrombosis (arterial or venous)
Hypertension
Gout
Peptic ulceration

half-life of 14 days. A single dose is usually effective for 2 years. It is, however, associated with an increased risk of leukaemic conversion.

Thrombosis and haemorrhage are common and vascular accidents are a common cause of death. Median survival time is 10–16 years and is similar with all treatments. Transition to myelofibrosis occurs in 30% and to acute leukaemia in 5% of patients.

12.9.2 Essential Thrombocythaemia

Overproduction of platelets leads to a sustained increase in platelet count above 400×10^9/l and often $> 1 \times 10^{10}$/l. Recurrent haemorrhage and thrombosis are the principal clinical features. Splenic enlargement is frequent but splenic atrophy due to platelet occlusion of the splenic microcirculation may also be seen. Abnormally large platelets are seen in the blood film and the marrow is similar to that seen in polycythaemia rubra vera. The condition must be distinguished from other causes of raised platelet count such as haemorrhage, iron deficiency and chronic infections.

When the platelet count is above 1000×10^9/l **hydroxyurea** or **interferon**-α is used to reduce the count to $< 500 \times 10^9$/l because of the increased risk of arterial occlusion in older patients. ^{32}P is suitable for some elderly patients who cannot attend for regular outpatient surveillance. Aspirin (150–300 mg daily) is indicated following thrombosis.

Patients have a very good outlook and rarely transform.

12.9.3 Myelofibrosis

In this condition there is an increase in circulating stem cells associated with the establishment of extramedullary haemopoiesis. There is reactive fibrosis in the marrow with stimulation of fibroblasts. Patients present with anaemia, massive splenomegaly, weight loss and bone pain. A leuco-erythroblastic blood film is found and the red cells show characteristic 'tear-drop' appearance. Anaemia, raised (or low) white cell and platelet counts are common. Bone marrow aspirate is not usually possible but trephine biopsy shows a hypercellular marrow with increased collagen deposition.

Treatment is supportive with blood transfusions, iron and folic acid but patients with gross myeloproliferation should be treated with cytotoxic agents such as hydroxyurea. Splenic irradiation may be useful to reduce myeloproliferation and occasionally splenectomy is considered when transfusion requirements are very high, when the spleen is causing distressing symptoms due to its size or when there is severe thrombocytopenia causing recurrent haemorrhage.

Transformation to acute leukaemia occurs in 10–20% of patients.

FURTHER READING

Gautier M, Cohen HJ. Multiple myeloma in the elderly. *J Am Geriatr Soc* 1994; 42:653–664.

Goldman JM. Treatment of chronic leukaemia: some topical questions. *Baillières Clin Haematol* 1997; 10:405–421.

Hoffbrand AV, Pettit JE. *Essential Haematology.* Blackwell Science, Oxford, 1993.

Mansouri A, Lipschitw DA. Myelodysplastic syndromes in the elderly. *J Am Geriatr Soc* 1992; 40:386–391.

Ossenkoppele GJ. Treatment of multiple myeloma in elderly patients. New developments. *Drugs Aging* 1997; 11:152–164.

Quaglino D, Furia N, Di Leonardo G et al. Therapeutic management of haematological malignancies in elderly patients. Biological and clinical considerations. Part 1. Myelodysplasias and the acute leukaemias. *Aging* 1997; 9:231–240.

Samson D. Multiple myeloma: current treatment. *Postgrad Med J* 1994; 70:404–410.

Chapter 13

Dermatological Disorders

13.1 PRESSURE SORES

Pressure sores (syn. pressure ulcers, decubitus ulcers) are highly prevalent in the elderly hospitalized population and in elderly people in nursing homes. They represent one of the most serious dermatological clinical problems in elderly people and are an important cause of secondary morbidity and mortality. The incidence and prevalence of pressure sores increase markedly with advancing age. In 1991, the incidence of pressure sores varied from 4 to 10% of all patients admitted to British district general hospitals, the incidence varying with case-mix and predictably increasing in older, frailer patients. The estimated cost of treating pressure sores in average-sized district general hospitals in the UK is £340 000 (1994 figures). This does not include the cost of additional visits by the district nurses, which is estimated at £100 000–£200 000. The current estimated lowest annual cost of treating pressure sores is £180 million in the UK and $3 billion in the USA.

Pressure sores are graded 1–4 in severity (Table 13.1; Plates I–IV), and severity will determine the patient's treatment. There are various ways of measuring pressure sore depth and extent, but probably the most useful is by means of serial instant colour photographs, which also provide a very useful method of assessing treatment efficacy. Nowadays, most pressure sores should be preventable in hospitals and nursing homes,

Table 13.1 Staging of pressure ulcers

Grade 1: Non-blanchable skin erythema
Grade 2: Breakdown of epidermis and part of dermis, but not subcutaneous tissue
Grade 3: Ulceration penetrates full skin thickness to fascia
Grade 4: Ulceration extending to involve muscle and bone tissue

Table 13.2 The Norton Scale for assessing risk of pressure ulcers

	Score			
Domain	4	3	2	1
Physical status	Good	Fair	Poor	Very poor
Mental status	Alert	Apathetic	Confused	Stupor
Activity	Ambulant	Walks with help	Chairbound	Bedbound
Mobility	Full	Slightly limited	Very limited	Immobile
Incontinence	None	Occasional (<2/day)	Usually urine	Double

Score <15 indicates significant risk, <12 indicates high risk.
Adapted from Norton D, McLaren R, Exton-Smith AN. *An Investigation of Geriatric Nursing Problems in Hospital*. Churchill Livingstone, Edinburgh, 1975.

with the use of pressure sore risk assessment scales, such as the Norton Scale (Table 13.2). Patients at high risk or those with established pressure sores should be nursed in specially designed pressure-relieving mattresses and seats, of which there is a wide variety for different circumstances. Skin may become devitalized in as short a time as 1 hour from unrelieved axial pressure four to six times that of the systolic blood pressure. Shearing forces and excess moisture on the skin (e.g. urinary incontinence) also contribute to the development of pressure sores. Therefore, the best preventive is a state of vigilance among nursing and medical staff, particularly if the patient's general condition deteriorates. Pressure and friction may be minimized in various ways, as outlined in Table 13.3.

Table 13.3 Pressure relief for pressure ulcer prevention and treatment

(1) Regular repositioning by nursing staff, e.g. 2-hourly turning in lateral decubitus posture, 30° foot-up tilt technique (to transfer pressure from pelvic bony prominences to gluteal muscles).
(2) Cushion, pillow or sheepskin protection of vulnerable bony prominences, heels.
(3) Pressure reducing mattress, e.g. silicone fibre mattress overlay (Spenco) for stage 1 and 2 pressure sores, alternating pressure mattress (Pegasus Airwave or Nimbus systems) for stage 2 and 3 pressure sores, low air-loss bed (Mediscus or Kinnair systems) or air fluidized bed (Clinitron) for stage 3 and 4 pressure sores.
(4) Pressure-reducing seating for patients who lack sensation or who cannot shift their weight, e.g. air-filled cellular cushion (Roho), contoured foam.

The principles of management of the pressure sore itself are as follows:

(i) **Remove the cause of excessive skin pressure** if possible, e.g. inappropriately hard seating in the case of an immobile patient, and ensure pressure relief of damaged area of skin.

(ii) **Remove necrotic tissue**, particularly if infected, by local debridement if necessary.

(iii) **Treat infection of surrounding soft tissue and bone** with systemic antibiotics if confirmed microbiologically or radiologically. **Avoid routine swabbing** of pressure ulcers, since cultures often reveal a mixed growth of organisms that has little or no clinical significance. Therefore, only take swab cultures when there is clinical evidence of infection spreading to surrounding living tissue. Until microbiological confirmation, suitable empirical antibiotic therapy is ceftazidime 1 g twice a day intravenously or ciprofloxacin 500 mg twice daily; metronidazole 400–800 mg twice daily may be added if there is strong suspicion of anaerobic infection. **Avoid use of topical antibiotics** (risk of causing bacterial antibiotic resistance and sensitization) and **most antiseptics**, which may inhibit granulation and wound healing.

(iv) **Remove slough** using gentle irrigation with sterile normal saline and non-astringent desloughing agents that do not impair wound healing to cover the wound surface, such as hydrogels (e.g. Intrasite Gel) if there is mild exudate or alginate-based materials (e.g. Sorbsan) if there is moderate to heavy exudate; enzymatic desloughing agents (e.g. streptokinase, streptodornase, collagenase) seldom significantly enhance other desloughing techniques, are expensive and by themselves are not very effective.

(v) **Keep the wound surface moist and occluded** from the atmosphere a much as possible. This means wound occlusion with hydrocolloids (e.g. Granuflex), hydrogels (e.g. Intrasite), transparent membranes (e.g. Micropore) or foam dressings (e.g. Lyofoam). Granuflex is easy to apply and is self-adhesive to surrounding healthy skin.

(vi) **Remove wound dressings as little as possible**. Frequent dressing changes (except where there is much exudate with overflow onto healthy skin) are to be avoided, since each dressing change inhibits granulation and epithelialization by mechanical disruption and desiccation.

(vii) **Treat underlying systemic problems aggressively**, e.g. hypotension, dehydration, anaemia, infection, malnutrition and vitamin deficiency.

Foul-smelling pressure sores result from heavy contamination of slough and necrotic tissue with anaerobic bacteria. If there are signs of infection of surrounding tissues, systemic antibiotic therapy with metronidazole is usually effective. The odour itself is controlled by use of an **activated charcoal dressing** (e.g. Actisorb Plus). If there is a large amount of exudate, an absorbent foam dressing with a charcoal backing is helpful (e.g. Lyofoam C). Other measures such as nursing the patient in a single room with good ventilation and air fresheners are also useful. **Black hard eschar** (most commonly on the heels) should be covered with dry gauze or thin layers or hydrocolloid (e.g. **Granuflex Extra Thin**), and not debrided if 'clean and dry'. As soon as the eschar begins to separate from underlying tissue, sloughing and exudate are common, and are best managed using a hydrocolloid (e.g. Granuflex) or hydrogel (e.g. Intrasite) dressing combined with mechanical heel protection.

Sacral, gluteal and trochanteric pressure sores are the most prevalent types of pressure ulcer in the elderly hospitalized or nursing home patient, and there is high risk of faecal and urinary contamination of such wounds. Close attention must be paid to controlled evacuation of bowel (with rectal enemas or suppositories) and bladder (with temporary urinary catheter) in bedbound patients. Also, the wound must be well covered and sealed, and for this purpose, hydrocolloid dressings cut to the shape of the sacral area and buttocks, and held in position with tape at the margins, are very useful.

Many hospitals and health care services now offer specialist wound care, usually delivered by a nurse specializing in tissue viability. Such expertise, if available, is invaluable in implementing high quality, evidence-based practice in pressure ulcer treatment and prevention.

13.2 CHRONIC LEG ULCERATION

Chronic leg ulceration occurs mostly commonly in elderly people, especially women. The pathophysiology is diverse, but usually results from chronic lower limb deep venous insufficiency, usually as a result of previous deep venous thrombosis, or from a combination of venous and arterial insufficiency (Plate V). Also, undetected arterial insufficiency may be the reason for failure of chronic venous ulcers to heal fully. The other common cause of chronic leg ulceration is diabetes mellitus (through a combination of small vessel disease, sensory neuropathy and sepsis). Rarely, ulcers are caused by vasculitis or local malignancy. Many patients have developed the post-phlebitic limb syndrome prior to manifesting venous ulceration, i.e. pitting oedema, haemosiderin pigmentation, lipodermatosclerosis and/or atrophy blanche. Venous ulcers are often precipitated by minor trauma and usually occur on the medial aspect of the distal one-third of the calf, often around the medial malleolus. Chronic indolent infection is common. A minority of venous ulcers results from pure superficial venous insufficiency (varicose veins) with intact, competent deep veins. These ulcers tend to be less severe and heal quickly with compression. Arterial ulcers are usually smaller than venous ulcers, and often occur in the toes or dorsum of the foot. There are usually symptoms and signs of chronic arterial insufficiency and often evidence of concurrent systemic arterial occlusive disease (e.g. ischaemic heart disease, cerebrovascular disease). Pedal pulses are usually absent or diminished, the foot is cold, capillary filling is sluggish and a reduced ankle/brachial Doppler index is detected, i.e. <1.0. A posterior tibial artery systolic pressure >100 mmHg and an ankle/brachial index >0.7 indicate that the leg's perfusion is sufficient for healing. Diabetic ulcers result from the arterial insufficiency, micro-angiopathy or peripheral neuropathy or a combination of these factors. Neuropathic ulcers are classically found over pressure points in the foot and ankle (e.g. over metatarsal heads, malleoli) and are painless.

The principles of **chronic venous leg ulcer** management are similar to pressure ulcer management, i.e. debridement, desloughing, control of infection, occlusive dressings and treatment of underlying disorders that contribute to poor wound healing. However, chronic venous leg ulcers usually require compression bandaging and mobilization of the ankle joint to promote the calf muscle pump and enhanced venous return. **Multi-layer bandages**, usually four-layer, are currently recommended. This consists of an inner protective layer, followed by a non-adhesive dressing, followed by an absorbent layer (e.g. cotton wool) and an outer compression layer (e.g. Tensopress). The bandage should give sustained graduated compression which is higher at the ankle than at the calf.

Bandages must be comfortable and firm, but never tight, and the outer layer must not be allowed to roll so as to avoid any ligature effect, which is detrimental. A fifth stockingette layer may be helpful to prevent this happening. Ankle movement must not be restricted and the patient should be encouraged to elevate the limb when not mobile. Bandages should be changed no more frequently than weekly, if possible, although severe ulcers with a large volume of exudate may require dressing and bandaging more frequently than this. Where the deep venous system is intact, surgical ligation of superficial varices may prevent recurrence of venous leg ulcers, but is of doubtful value in cases of combined superficial and deep venous insufficiency. Where there is concurrent deep venous occlusion and superficial varices, ligation of the latter may actually be detrimental.

Recurrence of venous ulceration may be prevented by leg elevation and use of a knee-length graded elastic compression stocking plus exercise where possible. If the leg is traumatized in the medial distal gaiter area (even trivially), prompt treatment of the lesion and temporary compression bandaging are helpful. Occasionally, chronic venous leg ulcers that fail to heal with conservative measures (particularly if overlying bony prominences) require pinch or split-thickness skin grafting.

Dermatitis secondary to topical medicaments ('**medicament dermatitis**'), e.g. lanolin and preservatives; (Plate VI) and so-called '**varicose eczema**' (syn. stasis eczema, gravitational eczema) occur in legs affected by venous hypertension. Patients usually have typical stigmata of long-standing venous hypertension with an overlying or surrounding vesiculopapular rash that is often intensely itchy. Patch testing may be helpful with identifying allergic contact hypersensitivity to topical medicaments, so that culprit medicaments can be avoided in the future. Bandaging or compression stocking combined with 0.025% betamethasone ointment (e.g. Betnovate RD) is usually effective.

With **arteriopathic leg ulcers**, revascularization is usually required for effective healing. This may be relatively simple with balloon angioplasty if a discrete proximal arterial stenosis with good radiographic 'run-off' is found at angiography. Elderly patients often tolerate vascular reconstructive surgery well, and operation should be considered if the patient is fit for general anaesthesia. Occasionally, conservative treatment is successful if sufficient collateral arterial blood supply develops or an important causative factor is eliminated (e.g. beta-blockers or drugs resulting in marked systemic hypotension). Recurrent arterial occlusion may be prevented by controlling risk factors for arterial occlusive disease (e.g. smoking, diabetes mellitus, hypertension, hyperlipidaemia). Vasodilator drugs are not recommended in these patients, whether ulceration is present or not. If there are signs of gangrene, amputation followed by prosthetic limb rehabilitation may be the most appropriate management for legs with deteriorating arterial ulceration.

Diabetic leg ulcers usually improve with optimal diabetic control, eradication of infection and removal of devitalized tissue (see also section 6.1.7). So-called '**total contact casting**' has been shown to facilitate healing in neuropathic ulceration. The ulcer is first debrided and soaked in povidone–iodine for 10 minutes. A hydrocolloid dressing that fits the shape of the ulcer with a 2 cm margin (to avoid leakage of exudate, slough) is then applied over the ulcer surface and secured with light adhesive tape at the edges. With minimal padding, a cast extending from the toes to below the knee joint level is then closely fitted, and a rocker heel level with the pretibial border is attached to the plantar surface of the cast. The rocker heel distributes vertical forces evenly over the foot and minimizes shear stress on the ulcer.

13.3   CELLULITIS AND INTERTRIGO

After respiratory and urinary tract infection, **cellulitis** is the third major cause of sepsis in old age. Cellulitis is a common disorder in elderly people since it usually occurs in people prone to chronic lower limb oedema and lymphoedema, disorders that occur mostly in middle and old age. Following one episode, patients are at increased risk of further attacks of cellulitis due to inflammatory damage of lymphatics. The portal of entry of infecting organisms may be trivial, e.g. superficial abrasion, insect bite, focus of dermatophytosis. The infecting organism is usually Group A haemolytic *Streptococcus* or infrequently, *Staphylococcus aureus*. There are no reliable laboratory tests for identifying the infecting organism quickly and accurately, unless there is associated suppuration, in which case aspiration or swabbing of pus will usually result in microbiological identification. When a site of origin (e.g. abrasion, ulcer) for the cellulitis is present, pathogens may be isolated

Table 13.4   Management of cellulitis

(a) Antibiotics
Severely unwell: benzylpenicillin 2 megaunits plus flucloxacillin 500 mg 6-hourly
intravenously
Mildly unwell: phenoxymethylpenicillin 500 mg plus flucloxacillin 500 mg 6-hourly
by mouth

(b) Analgesics
Opioids 4–6-hourly

(c) Emollients
Aqueous cream BP twice daily

(d) Elevation (to clear oedema) and exposure (to relieve burning sensation)

in about one-third of cases. Blood cultures are also worthwhile if the
patient is systemically unwell. The management of cellulitis is detailed
in Table 13.4.

Intertrigo refers to inflammation in the skin creases, most commonly in
the inguinal areas. It may also occur in submammary (Plate VII), natal
cleft, periumbilical, neck and axillary skin folds. The cause in most
cases is a combination of obesity and poor hygiene, but factors such as
diabetes mellitus and incontinence may be important also. Candidal
infection is usually present and a combination of a topical imidazole
(e.g. clotrimazole 1% or miconazole 2%) and a low-potency corticosteroid (e.g. hydrocortisone 1%) is usually curative. Canesten HC and
Daktacort are suitable preparations applied twice daily until the rash has
cleared.

13.4   XEROSIS AND PRURITUS

The ageing process itself commonly causes **xerosis** (dry skin), which is
the most prevalent cause of pruritus in the absence of primary skin
disorders. Xerosis is believed to be the result of age-related reduced
production of sebum, the natural skin moisturizing substance. Xerosis
may advance from a dry, scaling skin with marked desquamation to
frank eczema (**asteatotic eczema**), where there is intense drying and
fissuring of the skin, particularly on the pretibial and dorsal hand areas.

The latter appearance is often seen in frail, hospitalized elderly and is partly due to low ambient humidity, excessive bathing and increased use of soap. Xerosis is best managed with non-sensitizing topical emollients (e.g. aqueous cream BP three to four times daily), emollient bath additives (e.g. Bath E45), limited use of non-medicated soap in the genital and axillary areas and in more severe cases, with associated **asteatotic eczema**, low-potency topical corticosteroids (e.g. 1% hydrocortisone ointment). Lanolin-based emollients should be avoided in patients with frank asteatotic eczema because of the risk of sensitization and worsening of pruritus.

Scabies is a frequent cause of intense pruritus in old people with poor hygiene and self-care. It may elude diagnosis in some cases because the nodular rash has become chronic, or the classical burrowing tracks made by the sarcoptic mites are not evident clinically. Skin scrapings from skin lesions sometimes do not show the mites under light microscopy. However, a pruritic rash affecting the groins and genitalia should alert suspicion, particularly if pruritus is intense with increased skin temperature, e.g. in bed at night-time. More than one elderly person or staff member in the hospital or institutional care setting with a spreading, itching nodular rash of recent onset should also be treated as likely scabies. The treatment of choice is **permethrin 5%** applied to the whole skin surface (including head, neck, face and scalp), and washed off 12–24 hours later. Complete change and laundering of clothing and bedding are essential to ensure extermination of all mites, and many dermatologists recommend a second all-over skin application of permethrin 1 week after the initial treatment to further reduce the risk of relapse. Persons in close contact with the patient should be treated also. Despite effective destruction of the population of mites, the pruritus often persists for several days, sometimes up to 12 weeks after the scabicidal treatment, and a sedating antihistamine given at bedtime (e.g. chlorpheniramine 4 mg) may reduce intense pruritus and the risk of excoriative skin damage.

Generalized pruritus may be associated with a variety of systemic conditions, including iron deficiency anaemia, chronic renal failure, chronic biliary obstruction, diabetes mellitus, hypo- and hyperthyroidism, polycythaemia, lymphoma and carcinomatosis. Despite treatment for the underlying condition, symptomatic control of the pruritus may be difficult. Use of antihistamines in elderly patients may be limited by their tendency to oversedate and cause confusion (many antihistamines are also powerfully anticholinergic). In resistant cases, short courses of ultraviolet B therapy may be helpful.

13.5 HERPES ZOSTER ('SHINGLES')

Herpes zoster is a common problem in older people, the annual incidence rising from 5.1/1000 in people in their fifties to 10.1/1000 in octogenarians, possibly the result of age-related impaired cell-mediated immunity. In 4–5% of cases, the attack is recurrent. The pathophysiology is that of a severe dermal vasculitis, with ischaemic necrosis of skin and neural tissue, often followed by scarring and anaesthesia/neuralgia of the affected area which develops into eschar after 12–14 days. Typically, it occurs as a vesiculobullous eruption in a dermatomal distribution (Plate VIII). In the acute stages, pain may be intense and there is a risk of secondary bacterial infection of the damaged skin area. Ophthalmic herpes zoster, where the rash affects the ophthalmic division of the trigeminal nerve, often causes conjunctivitis and sometimes uveitis and keratitis. Secondary acute glaucoma can develop in those patients with uveitis.

The management of acute herpes zoster is summarized in Table 13.5. Corticosteroids are no better than placebo in acute herpes zoster for reducing the risk of postherpetic neuralgia. Newer antiviral drugs, such as famciclovir and valaciclovir (a prodrug of aciclovir), do not appear to be any more efficacious than aciclovir, although their three times per day dosing regimen may be an advantage where compliance is a concern with aciclovir (given five times daily). For exposed areas of skin, saline-soaked gauze is appropriate, whilst affected skin areas that are normally covered may be treated with a hydrocolloid dressing (e.g. Granuflex) or hydrogel (e.g Intrasite) with a polyurethane film covering. Secondary **local bacterial infection** may be treated with **topical framycetin** 1.5% or **mupirocin** 2% for 7–10 days. However, if the patient is systemically unwell or febrile, it is best to give oral or intravenous flucloxacillin 500 mg 6-hourly in combination with intravenous aciclovir. Herpes zoster in immunocompromised patients usually requires intravenous aciclovir therapy at a dose of 10 mg/kg 8-hourly.

The principal concern with herpes zoster infection in older people is development of **postherpetic neuralgia (PHN)**. Unfortunately, no

Table 13.5 Management of acute herpes zoster

(a) Simple analgesia
Paracetamol or opioids *regularly*

(b) Limit virus-mediated tissue damage
Aciclovir 800 mg five times daily orally (or intravenously if severe systemic upset); only of value if started within 72 hours of onset of rash or within 48 hours of appearance of last vesicle. Continue treatment until 48 hours after appearance of last lesion.

current treatment reliably prevents postherpetic neuralgia. Pain control in established PHN is often difficult. However, **tricyclic antidepressants** with noradrenaline reuptake inhibitory effects (e.g. amitriptyline, maprotiline, desipramine) are often helpful; interestingly, selective serotonin reuptake inhibitors (SSRIs) are not effective for PHN. Amitriptyline may be tried first at a starting dose of 10–25 mg nocte. Maprotiline and desipramine may be tried if patients are intolerant of anticholinergic side-effects from amitriptyline. **Mexiletine**, with its local anaesthetic properties, and **anticonvulsants** (e.g. **carbamazepine** or **sodium valproate**) at similar doses used to suppress seizure activity are suitable second-line drugs for PHN. Neuroleptics are of doubtful value, with the possible exception of chlorprothixene, which was effective in one uncontrolled study and did not cause significant extrapyramidal symptoms at doses up to 45 mg/day. **Transcutaneous electrical nerve stimulation (TENS)** may be worth trying, but firm evidence for its efficacy is lacking. Topical agents, such as **capsaicin** or **Emla** (a mixture of lignocaine 2.5% and prilocaine 2.5%), sometimes give relief where other treatments have failed, but the effect is short-lived. Resistant PHN can be treated by **sympathetic block** or local anaesthetic/corticosteroid injection of the affected nerve root. Surgical neurolysis of the dorsal root spinal canal entry zone may be offered in cases of unremitting, severe PHN if the patient is surgically fit.

13.6 MISCELLANEOUS DERMATOLOGICAL CONDITIONS OF OLD AGE

Seborrhoeic dermatitis is commonly seen in older people. It principally affects the head and neck, causing a desquamating, erythematous sometimes confluent eruption around the eyebrows, nasolabial folds, ears and scalp margin. It may also affect the presternal, inguinal, axillary and natal cleft areas. It is usually seen in neglected and frail elderly people, and may also be a feature of Parkinsonism, alcoholism and other neuropsychiatric conditions where the patient is unable to attend to adequate self-hygiene. *Pityrosporum orbiculare* has recently been implicated in the pathogenesis of seborrhoeic dermatitis. The management is with wet soaks to soften and remove crusts, emollients (e.g. aqueous cream) and 1% hydrocortisone cream. Topical clotrimazole 1% with or without 1% hydrocortisone (e.g. Canesten HC) may be applied to areas of skin where dermatitis is recurrent. Scalp seborrhoeic dermatitis may be treated with 2% ketoconazole shampoo (Nizoral) twice weekly for 2–4 weeks. Seborrhoeic blepharitis usually responds to 1% hydrocortisone cream.

Idiopathic dermatitis (eczema) occurs commonly in old people. It may affect any part of the integument, usually the extremities. Typically, there is an itchy, papular eruption that is often excoriated and lichenified. Lesions may vesiculate and become secondarily infected. Hydrocortisone 1% or 2.5% is the mainstay of treatment. Irritant substances like certain soaps and detergents should be avoided, as well as direct contact of the skin with woollen fabrics.

Seborrhoeic keratoses are usually seen in old people. They are usually pigmented and most often seen on the trunk and neck. They typically feel greasy to palpation and it is usually possible to peel them from the underlying skin surface with a wooden spatula. Occasionally, they are traumatized and bleed, but generally do not cause symptoms other than unsightliness. Sometimes, patients are concerned about melanoma, and firm reassurance can usually be given, but where there is doubt, excision biopsy of the lesion is advisable. Seborrhoeic keratoses are not pre-malignant.

Neurodermatitis (circumscribed lichen simplex) is a well-demarcated lichenified dermatitis which is not due to either external irritants or identified allergens. An initial pruritic stimulus generates an itch–scratch–itch cycle, which in turn causes lichenification (reactive epidermal hyperplasia). Lesions are usually seen in exposed areas, such as the forearms, legs and neck. Treatment is with topical corticosteroids and emollients. Occlusive dressings or bandages may be necessary to protect the affected skin from scratch trauma. Bandages impregnated with ichthymol (e.g. Ichthopaste) applied weekly may be particularly helpful with clearing the lesion.

Tinea infections are common in elderly people, possibly as a result of age-related reduction in dermal cell-mediated immunity. Inguinal (tinea cruris) and axillary areas, scalp and feet (tinea pedis) are commonly affected (Plate IX). There is usually a confluent erythematous, scaly, pruritic rash that is sometimes secondarily infected with *Candida* or Gram-positive cocci. Diagnosis is confirmed from skin scrapings and treatment consists of a topical imidazole (e.g. clotrimazole 1%) applied two to three times daily.

Toenail problems are common in old age, principally **onychexis** (upward thickening of the nail plate), **onychogryphosis** (forward over-growth of the nail plate) and **onychomycosis** (fungal nail infections). These disorders often cause discomfort and should be referred to a chiropodist for treatment. Nail scrapings should be sent for microbiological analysis in suspected fungal infection, and confirmed cases treated with oral **terbinafine** at a dose of 250 mg daily for 2 months (fingernails) or 3 months (toenails). An alternative is topical amorolfine 5% once–twice weekly for 9–12 months, but compliance may be a problem. Terbinafine and itraconazole have largely replaced griseofulvin in the treatment of dermatophytosis. Relapse rates are high in fungal nail infections, so repeat treatments are often necessary.

Bullous pemphigoid is the most common blistering eruption in old people. It causes a chronic vesiculobullous eruption that usually spares the mucous membranes and does not usually result in scarring. It is similar to **pemphigus vulgaris**, another autoimmune skin disorder, which usually involves mucous membranes. These two disorders may be differentiated clinically by Nikolsky's sign (induction of a blister by lateral skin pressure) which is positive in pemphigus vulgaris and negative in bullous pemphigoid. Also, blisters in pemphigus tend to be flaccid whilst those in cases of pemphigoid are usually tense (Plate X). Immunofluorescence studies of skin biopsies will accurately diagnose and distinguish the two similar conditions. Treatment of pemphigoid and pemphigus is with oral corticosteroids (starting dose 1 mg/kg daily for pemphigoid, 2.5 mg/kg daily for pemphigus). The disease usually remits after 12–18 months' therapy. Appropriate measures to minimize steroid-induced osteoporosis must be taken at the outset of therapy (see section 8.8). Involvement of conjunctival and oral mucous membranes should be treated with additional topical corticosteroids (e.g. triamcinolone 0.1% paste two to four times daily for mouth ulcers; betamethasone 0.1% ointment two to four times daily for conjunctival ulcers).

Erythroderma is an uncommon, but severe and potentially life-threatening generalized skin eruption that results in widespread erythema, scaling and oedema (Plate XI). It has a varied aetiology, most commonly resulting from drugs (e.g. gold, phenytoin, allopurinol, sulphonamides) and underlying psoriasis, seborrhoeic dermatitis, lymphoma or leukaemia. Hospitalization is usually required for rehydration and intensive skin care with emollients and topical high-potency corticosteroids. Systemic corticosteroids may be required in severe cases and broad-spectrum antibiotics if there are signs of secondary bacteraemia.

Cutaneous drug eruptions occur most commonly in elderly people, possibly because elderly people consume more drugs than any other age stratum. Virtually all drugs are capable of causing skin rashes of one type or another, most commonly urticarial, erythematous, purpuric and maculopapular. **Urticarial** eruptions usually occur 3–7 days after starting therapy, usually penicillins, aspirin, phenothiazines, tetracyclines and sulphonamides. Purpura commonly occurs as a result of treatment with corticosteroids (Plate XII) and may be severe when combined with age-related dermal atrophy in old people. It may also occur with any severe drug eruption where there is widespread capillary damage, as well as with idiosyncratic drug-induced bone marrow suppression (e.g. carbimazole, gold). Idiosyncratic **photosensitive eruptions** occur from exposure to a variety of drugs, such as thiazides, phenothiazines and sulphonylureas. **Fixed drug eruptions** occur in the same skin area and have the same skin effects each time the patient is exposed to the causative agent. Common examples include penicillins, aspirin and sulphonamides. Apart from stopping the offending drug, treatment is symptomatic. Occasionally, severe drug eruptions (e.g. erythema multiforme, toxic epidermal necrolysis) occur that may be life-threatening and require intensive skin therapy. Commonly associated drugs include non-steroidal anti-inflammatory agents, sulphonamides, penicillins and anticonvulsants. Severe erythema multiforme may take up to 8 weeks to resolve and it is controversial whether any therapy hastens improvement, e.g. systemic corticosteroids. No clear benefit has been proven with corticosteroids and their use does carry the risk of overwhelming sepsis.

Squamous cell, **basal cell** and **melanoma skin cancer** are discussed in section 9.8.

FURTHER READING

Angle N, Bergan JJ. Chronic venous ulcer. *Br Med J* 1997; 314:1019–1023.

Buckley C, Rustin MHA. Management of irritable skin disorders in the elderly. *Br J Hosp Med* 1990; 44:24–32.

Charlton E. Neuropathic pain. *Prescriber J* 1993; 33:244–249.

Conlon CP. Herpes zoster. *Prescriber J* 1995; 35:46–52.

Cullum N, Deeks J, Fletcher A et al. The prevention and treatment of pressure sores. *Effective Health Care* 1995; 2:1–16.

Dealey C. *Managing Pressure Sore Prevention*. Mark Allen Publishing UK, Dinton, Wilts, 1997.

Kurban RS, Kurban AK. Common skin disorders of aging: diagnosis and treatment. *Geriatrics* 1993; 48:30–42.

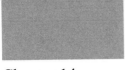

Chapter 14

Palliative Problems

14.1 CANCER-RELATED PAIN

The first principle of managing cancer pain is an adequate and full assessment of the cause of the pain. Over 80% of cancer pain can be controlled with the regular use of oral analgesics. Consideration must be given to treating the underlying cause of the pain by surgery, radiotherapy or chemotherapy and to the possibility that the pain may not be related to cancer.

14.1.1 Analgesic Drugs

The basic principle of pain relief in palliative care, based on the World Health Organization analgesic ladder, is that the choice of drug should be based on the severity of the pain and not the stage of the disease. Drugs should be administered in standard doses at regular intervals in a stepwise fashion (the analgesic ladder). If a non-opioid (e.g. paracetamol), or, in turn, a weak opioid (e.g. codeine) is not sufficient, a strong opioid is used. Either a strong or a weak opioid should be used, not both, and the non-opioid should generally be continued. Adjuvant analgesics may be added at any time (see below). This approach is valid in the elderly population but age-related changes in pharmacokinetics and pharmacodynamics of drugs mean that certain adaptations are necessary.

When a non-opioid drug is used with a weak opioid, combination formulations may be more convenient. Care must be taken with the dose of each drug in the formulation. For example, although co-codamol (codeine phosphate 8 mg, paracetamol 500 mg) and co-dydramol (dihydrocodeine tartrate 10 mg, paracetamol 500 mg) may be effective in many elderly patients, higher doses of codeine (30–60 mg 4- to 6-hourly) or dihydrocodeine (30 to 60 mg 4- to 6-hourly) should be tried first before moving on to stronger opioids if the pain is not controlled. Compound preparations with higher opioid doses include Solpadol or Tylex (codeine phosphate 30 mg, paracetamol 500 mg) and Remediene Forte (dihydrocodeine tartrate 30 mg, paracetamol 500 mg). An alternative is co-proxamol, which contains dextropropoxyphene 32.5 mg.

Strong Opioid Analgesics

Morphine is the most commonly used and its relatively short half-life of 2 to 4 hours makes it an appropriate choice in elderly patients who may be more sensitive to its analgesic (and toxic) effects. When possible it should be given by mouth, the dose titrated to abolish pain and doses repeated at 4-hourly intervals so that the pain is prevented from returning. There is no upper dose limit. A quick release formulation of morphine (e.g. **morphine elixir**) with a rapid onset and short duration of action is used for dose titration. The recommended method which is appropriate in elderly patients is to prescribe a regular 4-hourly dose (e.g. 5 mg) but allow extra doses for 'breakthrough pain' plus 10 mg nocte. After 24–48 hours the daily requirements are assessed and the regular doses adjusted as necessary. Although patients with advancing disease may require continual adjustment of dose many patients reach a period of stability where requirements remain the same over weeks or months. A once or twice daily preparation of controlled-release morphine is then used as a maintenance dose. Elderly patients are predisposed to accumulation of active morphine metabolites so if clinical toxicity occurs a switch to another opioid is warranted. Opioid alternatives to morphine are listed in Table 14.1.

Although the rectal route may be used if the patient is unable to take drugs by mouth, morphine suppositories are not very readily available and are of limited dose. For most patients it is more convenient to convert directly to a subcutaneous infusion using a syringe driver. The relative potency of opioids is increased when they are given parenterally and the total daily oral morphine dose should be halved if converting to subcutaneous morphine. If subcutaneous diamorphine is used only a third of the total morphine dose is needed. Rarely, patients may need intravenous administration.

Tolerance and addiction are rarely a problem in the clinical management of cancer pain. Sedation is common initially but usually resolves within

Table 14.1 Opioid alternatives to morphine

Drug	Comment
Hydromorphine	7 times as potent as morphine; short half-life so metabolites less likely to accumulate
Fentanyl	Self-adhesive patches changed every 72 hours; suitable for patients with stable pain; used with quick release oral opioid for breakthrough pain
Diamorphine	Prodrug of morphine; greater solubility confers an advantage over morphine for parenteral administration
Buprenorphine	Sublingual administration for patients needing low doses of opioids

a few days. Nausea may also be a problem at first and if it persists **metoclopramide** (10 mg three times a day) or **haloperidol** (1.5 mg nocte) are effective antiemetics. In all patients constipation should be pre-empted with stimulant laxatives. Dry mouth is a troublesome adverse effect for many patients and may be helped by frequent sips of cold water or sucking boiled sweets. Cognitive impairment is a particular problem in elderly patients who may be predisposed to this effect by concurrent disorders, such as dementia or metabolic disturbances or administration of other psychotropic drugs. If possible, therefore, non-essential drugs should be discontinued on starting strong opioids. Elderly patients with poor respiratory function should be observed closely while opioid therapy is instituted.

14.2 MANAGEMENT OF DIFFICULT PAIN PROBLEMS

14.2.1 Neuropathic Pain

Neuropathic pain may be produced by a tumour infiltrating or compressing neural tissue but may also be caused by surgery, radiotherapy, chemotherapy or viral infection. The pain is described as burning, stabbing, stinging or aching and may be superficial or deep. It may be precipitated by various stimuli including light touch or cold.

Table 14.2   Adjuvant analgesics for neuropathic pain

Drug	Indication
Corticosteroids (dexamethasone 8–16 mg/day)	Raised intracranial pressure Soft tissue infiltration Nerve compression
Tricyclic antidepressants (amitriptyline 10–150 mg)	Pain relief (independent of antidepressant effect) Nerve compression or infiltration Paraneoplastic neuropathies
Anticonvulsants (sodium valproate 200 mg twice daily, up to 1600 mg/day); carbamazepine 200 mg nocte, up to 400 mg twice daily)	Pain relief as for tricyclics; sodium valproate better tolerated than carbamazepine
Antiarrhythmics (mexiletine 50–300 mg three times daily)	Second/third-line when others have failed
NSAIDs	Bone pain Soft tissue infiltration Hepatomegaly

A trial of opioids is important, usually in conjunction with an adjuvant analgesic (Table 14.2). The latter are drugs whose primary indication is other than pain but which have an analgesic effect in some cases, e.g. corticosteroids, non-steroidal anti-inflammatory drugs (NSAIDs), tricyclic antidepressants, anticonvulsants and some antiarrhythmic drugs.

Transcutaneous electrical nerve stimulation (TENS) uses surface electrodes to stimulate large diameter nerves in the skin and subcutaneous tissues. Success depends on correct positioning of the electrodes and optimal adjustment of the electrical output. Only some patients benefit and efficacy tends to decline over a few weeks. Acupuncture, physiotherapy and occupational therapy may all help in certain patients.

14.2.2   Incident Pain

Incident pain is transient pain precipitated by a voluntary action, such as weight-bearing in patients with bony metastases, and can severely limit a patient's functional ability.

Management relies on treatment of the underlying cause if possible (such as radiotherapy for bony metastases) and optimization of the analgesic regimen with opioids and appropriate adjuvants. 'Breakthrough doses' of NSAIDs or opioids may be particularly useful. For some patients spinal administration of an opioid combined with a local anaesthetic may be useful, but requires specialist input. Physiotherapy and occupational therapy may help with mobilization and maintenance of muscle function. Spinal stabilization with surgery can relieve pain caused by vertebral destruction in otherwise reasonably fit patients with a prognosis of at least 3 months. Internal stabilization of a long bone or joint replacement may help patients even if they have advanced metastatic disease.

14.2.3 Visceral Pain

Visceral pain is often poorly localized and difficult to describe unless there is involvement of a somatically innervated structure such as the parietal peritoneum.

Management is initially with analgesics. However, invasive techniques such as coeliac axis block in patients with carcinoma of the pancreas or stomach should be considered at an early stage. Pelvic malignancies may be complicated by bladder and rectal tenesmus, severe perianal pain and severe rectal spasm such as proctalgia fugax. These pains respond poorly to opioids but smooth muscle relaxants, sedative drugs and anticholinergics may help. Perianal pain may respond to neurolytic saddle block.

14.2.4 Other Anaesthetic Techniques

Spinal opioids (with a local anaesthetic for incident pain) are indicated in patients with opioid responsive pain who have intolerable adverse effects when the drug is taken systemically at doses needed to control pain. Drugs may be delivered to the central nervous system via fine catheters placed within the epidural space or within the cerebrospinal fluid in the subarachnoid space. Catheters may be tunnelled subcutaneously to exit under the skin and are attached to a bacterial filter for intermittent or continuous drug administration. Alternatively, they can be connected to a subcutaneously implanted reservoir or pump delivery system. Infection and mechanical failure of the system are the commonest complications.

Invasive neurolytic procedures have declined in use because of improved pharmacological management but may provide excellent relief in selected patients. For example, coeliac plexus block can be useful for intractable pain arising from the pancreas and subarachnoid neurolysis can give relief to patients with perianal pain due to pelvic malignancy. Cordotomy lesions produced surgically or percutaneously by radio-frequency probe may provide excellent pain relief for unilateral somatic pain below the fifth cervical dermatome in patients whose survival prognosis is less than 9 months. However, sensory disturbance is an invariable accompaniment, and motor weakness and sphincter disturbances are common.

14.3 BREATHLESSNESS

Breathlessness is common during the terminal stages of cancer and is a particularly distressing symptom for both patients and their carers. While there is usually an obvious cause such as pleural effusion or extrinsic bronchial compression, in some patients no cause is found.

Management of a breathless patient should be individualized and often needs a multidisciplinary approach. Treatment will depend on the underlying cause and therapeutic options for specific situations are given in Table 14.3.

Oxygen is usually seen as a non-specific treatment for breathlessness and patients may become highly dependent on it. It is not clear at present which patients are most likely to benefit from oxygen and the advantages and disadvantages should be considered carefully for each individual (Table 14.4). The use of nasal cannulae can avoid some of the problems associated with oxygen masks and a 24-hour trial of oxygen with oximetry and subjective assessment by the patient may be very useful. In many patients a full explanation combined with the use of a bedside fan and anxiolytics may remove the need for oxygen. If long-

Table 14.3   Therapeutic options for management of breathlessness in specific situations

Pleural effusion
Pleural aspiration
Pleurodesis
Pleuroperitoneal shunt

Pericardial effusion
Aspiration ± fenestration

Hypoxia
Oxygen

Lymphangitis
High-dose corticosteroids (dexamethasone 16 mg/day)

Endobronchial disease
High-dose corticosteroids (dexamethasone 16 mg/day)
Laser therapy
Cryotherapy
Stenting

Table 14.4   Advantages and disadvantages of oxygen therapy

Potential advantages	Potential disadvantages
Reverses hypoxia Improved well-being Placebo effect	Ties patient to oxygen source Potential loss of respiratory drive Claustrophobia Difficulty in talking Dry mouth Cost

term oxygen is considered appropriate an oxygen concentrator rather than oxygen cylinders should be used.

Anxiolytics, particularly **benzodiazepines**, have a role in managing breathlessness even in patients who are not particularly anxious. Concerns about respiratory depression are usually unfounded and must be weighed against potential benefit. Some patients may experience severe panic attacks and feel that they are about to die. They should be advised about coping with these by relaxation techniques and deep breathing in addition to small doses of benzodiazepines. Choices of anxiolytics include lorazepam (0.5–2 mg) orally or sublingually for episodes of acute breathlessness, diazepam (5 mg initially) if a regular anxiolytic is required and midazolam (subcutaneously (2.5–5 mg) or by infusion (10 mg/24 hours initially)) if parenteral administration is required.

Low-dose oral opioids can improve breathlessness. The dose can be titrated in the same way as when used for pain control but lower doses and smaller increments should be used. As little as 2.5 mg of morphine elixir every 4 hours may be sufficient. If a patient is already taking controlled release morphine, it is sometimes beneficial to convert to a short-acting preparation and allow for a dose increment.

14.4 COUGH

Cough is common in malignant disease and may be productive (with the patient either able or not able to cough effectively) or non-productive. Simple measures such as a change in position at night may be very effective.

Cough suppressants are used to manage dry cough, or irritant nocturnal cough and cough in dying patients. The most effective agents are the opioids, with codeine linctus having a mild antitussive effect and the strong opioids having a more pronounced one.

Mucolytic treatments such as simple linctus or nebulized saline may help patients with retained bronchopulmonary secretions and an unproductive cough but are not suitable for patients unable to expectorate.

Nebulized local anaesthetics can relieve intractable, non-productive cough for which no other treatment has been found. Both lignocaine (up to 5 ml of 2% solution every 6 hours) and bupivacaine (up to 5 ml of 0.25% solution) have been used. Treatment reduces the sensitivity of the gag reflex so patients should not eat or drink for an hour afterwards. Bronchospasm can occur so nebulized bronchodilators should be available.

Dexamethasone (1–10 mg/day) is used to relieve cough related to endobronchial tumour, lymphangitis or radiation pneumonitis.

Many patients have increased airway secretions but are unable to cough. In these circumstances, it may be more appropriate to give **hyoscine**

hydrobromide by subcutaneous injection (0.2–0.4 mg) or by subcutaneous infusion over 24 hours (1.2–2.4 mg).

14.5 HAEMOPTYSIS CAUSED BY LUNG TUMOUR

It is important to establish that the blood has come from the chest and not the nose, upper respiratory or gastrointestinal tract. Radiotherapy and laser therapy are particularly effective at controlling minor bleeding from an endobronchial tumour, which may be treated initially with oral haemostatic agents such as tranexamic acid. Massive haemoptysis in the context of palliative care usually means that resuscitation is inappropriate and management is aimed at reducing awareness and fear with judicious use of opioids and benzodiazepines.

14.6 STRIDOR

Treatment with corticosteroids such as dexamethasone 16 mg daily can bring rapid relief but radiotherapy, endobronchial stent insertion or laser ablation (for intrinsic large airway obstruction) are other options to be considered.

14.7 NAUSEA AND VOMITING

Up to 60% of people with advanced cancer suffer from nausea, vomiting and/or retching. Common causes and treatment of vomiting patients with advanced cancer are listed in Table 14.5. Nausea can be treated with oral drugs but alternative routes (such as subcutaneous infusion) are needed for patients with severe nausea or vomiting.

14.8 DEHYDRATION

Frail elderly patients with poor venous access may be unable to take sufficient fluid orally for a variety of reasons, such as severe malaise, weakness, vomiting and gastrointestinal obstruction. Under such

Table 14.5 Common causes and specific treatment of vomiting in patients with advanced cancer

Cause	Treatment
Drugs	
Opioids	Metoclopramide, haloperidol
Chemotherapy	Dexamethasone
Gastric	
Gastritis/ulceration	Stop NSAID
	Omeprazole/H_2-receptor antagonist
Gastroduodenal obstruction	Metoclopramide, dexamethasone, hyoscine
Functional gastric stasis	Metoclopramide/domperidone/cisapride
Constipation	Laxatives, enemas
Biochemical	
Renal failure	Haloperidol
Hypercalcaemia	Rehydration, bisphosphonates
Infection	Antibiotics
Raised intracranial pressure	Dexamethasone (16 mg/day)
Vestibular disturbance	Cyclizine/hyoscine
Anxiety	Reassurance, anxiolytic drugs
Cough induced	Antitussive

circumstances administration of fluid subcutaneously rather than intravenously may be a simple and safer option. The technique of hypodermoclysis involves rehydrating a patient with isotonic fluids via the subcutaneous tissues. One to 2 litres are usually infused in a 24-hour period, but up to 3 litres can be infused by adding hyaluronidase to the infusion fluid. The advantages of hypodermoclysis are ease of administration, little pain, no requirement for a doctor to set it up and low incidence of infection. Normal (0.9%) saline is used in preference to 5% dextrose, which may be irritant when given subcutaneously. Supplemental potassium in the saline infusion is avoided for the same reason.

Table 14.6 Potentially reversible causes of fatigue and anorexia

Fatigue	Anorexia
Hypocortisolism	Nausea
Electrolyte imbalance	Constipation
Hypotension	Dry mouth
Drugs (opioids, antihypertensives)	Oro-oesophageal thrush

14.9 FATIGUE AND ANOREXIA

These symptoms are a major cause of concern for patients and their carers. Some causes are potentially reversible (Table 14.6) and should be treated. Other useful measures include dietetic and occupational therapy advice. Corticosteroids often have a potent but short-lived effect on appetite and dexamethasone 4 mg daily has less mineralocorticoid effect than prednisolone. Progestogens at high doses increase appetite and allow weight gain but because the effect is slow they are unsuitable for patients who only have weeks to live. Alcohol may also stimulate appetite.

FURTHER READING

Baines MJ. Nausea, vomiting, and intestinal obstruction. *Br Med J* 1997; 315:1148–1150.

Davis CL. Breathlessness, cough, and other respiratory problems. *Br Med J* 1997; 315:931–934.

Faull C. Symptom control in terminal illness. *Prescriber J* 1998; 38:32–39.

O'Neill B, Falon M. Principles of palliative care. *Br Med J* 1997; 315:801–804.

Regnard CBF, Davies A. *Symptom Relief in Advanced Disease*, 4th edn. Hachland & Hachland, Hale, Cheshire, 1998.

Sykes J, Johnson R, Hanks GW. Difficult pain problems. *Br Med J* 1997; 315:867–870.

Index

Index compiled by Anne McCarthy